CYCLE
MAGIC

CYCLE MAGIC

Your Guide to Align with
Natural Energy Cycles, Beat Burnout
and Manifest Your Dream Life

• • • • • • • • • •

ELLE SERAFINA
Creator of Cycle Magic®

HAY HOUSE
Carlsbad, California • New York City
London • Sydney • New Delhi

Published in the United Kingdom by:
Hay House UK Ltd, 1st Floor, Crawford Corner,
91–93 Baker Street, London W1U 6QQ
Tel: +44 (0)20 3927 7290; www.hayhouse.co.uk

Text © Elle Serafina LLC, 2026

Cover design: Kara Klontz
Interior design: Claudine Mansour Design
Interior photos/illustrations: Courtesy of the author

The moral rights of the author have been asserted.

All rights reserved. No part of this book may be reproduced by any mechanical, photographic or electronic process, or in the form of a phonographic recording; nor may it be stored in a retrieval system, transmitted or otherwise be copied for public or private use, other than for 'fair use' as brief quotations embodied in articles and reviews, without prior written permission of the publisher.

The information given in this book should not be treated as a substitute for professional medical advice; always consult a medical practitioner. Any use of information in this book is at the reader's discretion and risk. Neither the author nor the publisher can be held responsible for any loss, claim or damage arising out of the use, or misuse, of the suggestions made, the failure to take medical advice or for any material on third-party websites.

Tradepaper ISBN: 978-1-83782-610-0
E-book ISBN: 978-1-4019-9825-7
Audiobook ISBN: 978-1-4019-9826-4

10 9 8 7 6 5 4 3 2 1

This product uses responsibly sourced papers, including recycled materials and materials from other controlled sources. For more information, see www.hayhouse.co.uk

The authorized representative in the EU for product safety and compliance is Penguin Random House Ireland, Morrison Chambers, 32 Nassau Street, Dublin D02 YH68, Ireland. https://eu-contact.penguin.ie

Printed and bound by CPI Group (UK) Ltd, Croydon CR0 4YY

*Dedicated to my beloved grandmother Olive May,
and to you, dear reader.*

CONTENTS

Introduction   ix

PART I: From Misaligned to Miss Aligned   1

    Chapter 1   Are You Feeling Misaligned?   3
    Chapter 2   Cycle Basics   34
    Chapter 3   How Cycle Magic Works   46

PART II: The Cycle Magic System   53

    Chapter 4   Attune   55
    Chapter 5   Awaken   113
    Chapter 6   Thrive   166
    Chapter 7   Surrender   202
    Chapter 8   Cycle Mastery   249

Resources   264
References   267
About the Author   273
Acknowledgments   275

INTRODUCTION

Soul Calling

Just a few short years ago a series of unpleasant wake-up calls rocked me out of my comfort zone. At the time, I'd grown accustomed to living in struggle mode, even though it was exhausting and stressful. I believed that manifesting the life of my dreams would require a lot of physical and mental effort. But no matter how much I did, it was never enough, and it had started to feel like I wasn't enough. Despite my declining self-esteem, energy, thyroid function, social life, and bank account, the whispers of my soul still assured me that I was meant for more.

Fed up with feeling stuck, I planned a cozy night in for New Year's Eve to focus on designing my year ahead. I decided that the new year would be one of transformational wellness, opening up to love, shifting whatever was holding me back, and becoming a co-creator with the Universe to bring my heart and soul desires into manifestation.

As midnight drew closer, I lit candles and gathered my planner, markers, and laptop, feeling a subtle electrical current of excitement building. I began by revisiting the notes, voice memos, screenshots, saved posts, and Pinterest mood boards I'd compiled over the year about various goals and ideas I wanted to set in motion someday. As I sorted through file after file of workout routines, habit trackers, recipes, dating tips, decor palettes, self-care checklists, and entrepreneurial ideas, my excitement turned into anxiety. It was in that moment that I realized I was a collector of desires—plucked from the ether and filed away in an ever-expanding portfolio of dreams that might never come to fruition. In my scattered attempts at manifesting, I'd developed a habit of capturing and categorizing ideas but not *embodying* them. Countless notes and visuals wove together the tapestry of a dream life—money in the bank, time to spend in nature, a nourishing diet, abundant energy, creative hobbies, enriching social connections, fitness and vitality, exciting business ventures, and marriage to a man I could wear heels with. I sighed as the weight of all the potential versions of my future self rested like a heavy burden of unfulfilled wishes on my shoulders. It seemed as though it would take another *lifetime* for all of these things to line up.

I decided that I couldn't wait another lifetime. In that very second I gave myself permission to live with purpose—starting *now*. But how? While the world around me was based upon hustling, competing, and winning, I knew in my soul there was a better way for me. I didn't want to chase my dreams anymore. I wanted to attract them. I wanted to *align* with their energy. I decided that I'd have to approach this challenge with everything I had—mind, body, and soul.

The Magic of Cycles

In the weeks and months that followed, I began experimenting with ways to align with the universal energies that exist all around us, in nature and in our bodies. I took a deep dive into the menstrual cycle and feminine energy, and then integrated this knowledge with the metaphysical teachings I'd studied for more than a decade through the lenses of astrology, energy work, and spirituality. What I found was revolutionary.

I began tracking my menstrual cycle and the moon cycle and checking in with my body. When I first tuned in to my body, I often felt discomfort—tightness in my neck, jaw, and shoulders. I noticed myself rushing a lot and scrunching over my desk, and that my breathing was shallow. For the first time in a long time I was escaping my mind and feeling into the sensations in my body—and she felt like a stranger, not a reflection of my true self. Despite the initial discomfort, the insightful whispers from my body proved to be very valuable. I started to learn the times of day, week, and month when my energy peaked, and when it began to wane. I practiced conserving energy whenever I felt it dipping and maximizing it when it rose. I was able to recognize and anticipate the natural ebbs and flows of my energy, and this was truly a breakthrough. I no longer needed to consume caffeinated drinks or sugary snacks to get me through most days.

I'd always liked the idea of tracking my daily wellness habits but was burned out from feeling like a failure whenever I had to skip a day. I wanted to hold myself accountable for completing new goals and habits without trying to keep up with a long list of daily tasks. I decided instead to incorporate habit tracking on a monthly basis, aligning with the four phases of a cycle. This immediately felt more expansive.

I leveraged windows of time that were conducive to deepening intuition to crystallize my heart and soul desires into focus. I aligned my actions with uplifting energies to propel myself forward with ease, and I embraced contracting energies to delve into inner work and create small shifts in my mindset that resulted in big transformations in my external reality. I didn't know it then, but these experiments were the seedlings of an energy-centric system I would refine over the next months and years to consistently move me in the direction of my dreams.

Today, my life is aligned with the desires of my heart and soul, and I've been able to make all of my New Year's dreams a reality—and more! From the outside, it may seem as though it took a lot of effort to manifest my desires, but in truth it was a lot of fun. I leveraged natural energy cycles to move me through the phases of intentional action, reflection, planning, and creativity. It's an ongoing journey of co-creation with the Universe. Looking back now, I feel appreciation for the catalysts that led up to that turning point on New Year's Eve, as difficult as they were to confront at the time. I'm grateful that I've been able to continuously attract my desires into my life by aligning with natural energy cycles—and I know you can do this too!

Are you ready to create your own Cycle Magic?

Your Cycle Magic Journey

If, like me, you've been feeling burned out but know deep down that you're meant for more (even if you don't know exactly *what* that is), then this book will guide you to tap into your heart and soul desires. It will teach you to take aligned actions that will propel those seedlings into glorious blossoms, to start embodying your dream life now, and to explore the inner-work exercises that will help you align your vibration to attract the things you most desire. Then, you can usher your dreams into reality—without the hustle.

To align with these natural energy cycles, you *don't* have to:

- Think positive all the time
- Be spiritual
- Follow a strict routine
- Be constantly in sync
- Prepare anything in advance

- Know exactly what it is that you want right now
- Understand astrology, spirituality, physics, or energy
- Have a perfect menstrual cycle
- Have all the free time in the world

These energy cycles and rhythms will meet you where you're at so you can begin to gently align with them and allow them to support your manifesting journey.

Traditionally, women of cultures from all over the world have lived in accordance with the currents of natural energy cycles and rhythms such as menstrual and moon cycles, but this synchronization has been lost in our modern society. Instead, we contend with the 24-hour news cycle, the glorification of hyperproductivity, and the relentless demands of the daily grind. To keep up with the fast-paced changes of today, we tend to live in our minds, detached from the wisdom of our bodies and the intuitive guidance of our souls.

Our bodies, minds, and souls were not built for this kind of life. It's only in the past century or so—compared to our three hundred thousand years of existence—that we've increasingly had to navigate a proliferation of chemicals, processed foods, Wi-Fi signals, social media notifications, and countless other stressors our biology hasn't had time to adapt to. We are living in an era of evolutionary mismatch.[1] Everyday life has become a race to keep up with the constant demands on our time and attention, with seemingly no time to develop our passions and realize our deepest desires. This is especially true for women, because our hormones ebb and flow over the course of a month and yet we strive to meet the same fast pace every day. It is simply unsustainable. Anxiety affects almost 20 percent of U.S. adults, and depression is at an all-time high,[2] with women being twice as likely as men to be diagnosed with depression.[3] Estimates suggest that between 75 and 90 percent of doctor visits are stress-related.[4] Besides pushing our physical bodies beyond what they're capable of, many of us feel as though time is slipping away, and we don't know how to create a more fulfilling life without burning out. It's all so tiring! And it doesn't allow us to really live.

I call this phenomenon being "misaligned." We are living out of alignment with the natural energy cycles of our bodies and the Universe. But we all have the power, by making conscious choices, to impact our physical, mental, and spiritual wellness. We can even enhance and upregulate our genes through our lifestyle choices, thanks to the science of epigenetics. While there are forces in life that can keep us stuck if we get tangled up in them, the good news is that there are other powerful forces to align with to propel ourselves along a pathway toward living a life of wellness. In the chapters that follow, I outline the nature of these natural energy cycles and offer tools and exercises for how you can best align with them to reap the most benefits. You'll discover that there are four energetic phases of a cycle, which I've named Attune, Awaken, Thrive, and Surrender. Their names reflect the dominant energies available, and these four phases make up the Cycle Magic system, which you can align with each month either through your menstrual cycle or the moon cycle.

In Part I of Cycle Magic, we delve into natural energy cycles and rhythms, along with the obstacles that can prevent us from aligning with them. Shining a light on what may be holding us back can empower us to identify these forces, and then we can use the practices in Part II to navigate through them.

Each chapter in Part II includes exercises, tools, and practices to support you in manifesting your desires with ease and flow—almost as if you are bending time. By journeying through the four phases, you will not only identify the true desires of your heart and soul, but also equip yourself with the tools needed to take action on achieving them and begin living your fullest life. The Cycle Magic system is one you can use continually and adapt to your needs while you manifest your desires, whether they are related to your career, health, relationships, finances, lifestyle, or anything else. The more you practice this way of approaching your goals, the more you make it your own, and that's what true empowerment looks like.

The exercises for each phase can include guided meditations, activations, habit tracking, embodiment practices, journaling, immersion in nature, personal mantra creation, or workshops on topics like letting go, transforming limiting beliefs, and identifying boundaries. These exercises allow you to gain experience in working with natural energy cycles by going through the process of self-inquiry and activation. Each phase brings together a collection of practices that you can explore and revisit whenever the time feels aligned. They are not designed to be fully completed each month, but rather approached with flexibility and curiosity so you can try what speaks to you. This is *your* manifesting journey! It's time to escape the blueprint of "life happening to me" and become empowered to design the life that will *truly* bring you fulfillment. Let's align and create some magic!

PART I

FROM MISALIGNED TO MISS ALIGNED

Chapter 1

ARE YOU FEELING MISALIGNED?

• • • • • • • • • •

Deep within you lies a spark—a subtle voice or inner knowing—that whispers, "You are meant for more." Life, with all its busyness, often drowns out this voice. But every so often, it returns to remind you that there's a different way to live: one that's more aligned, expansive, and abundant.

You're about to embark on a beautiful journey filled with magic, empowerment, heart-centered practices, and soul-satisfying challenges that will excite you. But as we know, beautiful journeys don't always begin that way, do they? They often start somewhere amid a struggle.

We can become so deeply invested in striving and pursuing that the idea of letting go in favor of a different path fills us with uncertainty. We're accustomed to the relentless pace of day-to-day demands, and wish our bodies would keep up with our minds. Reaching the point at which aspiring diverges into tiring, we find ourselves tethered to the daily grind. Our spirit may seek rest and rejuvenation, but we've set such high expectations for our performance that there never seems to be a good time to retreat. People are counting on us. There's so much to achieve, and only so much success to go around. But might there be more to the story?

We don't need to sacrifice our autonomy by adhering to the limitations of the daily paradigm. The Cycle Magic system is an invitation to open up to a more expansive way of being. It's not about letting go of achievement, but rather about releasing the tight grip on our current living patterns that prevents us from receiving all the abundance that's available. I used to resist change, but I've come to realize that it's a necessary ingredient for a happy life. The clues are all around us in the constellations slowly shifting minute by minute, the snow giving way to blossoming wildflowers, and our perspectives evolving with each new book we read or conversation we have. We are not designed to remain static or constrained.

Living in misalignment with the flow of natural energy cycles can put our wellness at risk, contributing to physical exhaustion, emotional imbalance, and a sense of detachment from our true selves. If we continue in this way, it can lead to burnout, chronic stress, and a deeper disconnect from our purpose and potential. It's easy to overlook the subtle signs of misalignment, but change is inevitable. The Universe has a way of getting our attention by delivering gifts of transformation—invitations to experience a powerful metamorphosis into something greater. These shake-ups can alter the direction of our life and act as catalysts for positive change, urging us to realign and embrace a healthier, more balanced way of being. You'll recognize these gifts of transformation by their unexpected or unappealing packaging—at first, you might resist them, but once you unwrap their message, you'll see how empowering they can be. For me, these unwelcome gifts began to surface during the hap-hap-happiest season of all.

Gifts of Transformation

It was a bright and sunny Christmas morning in Los Angeles and Dad was in town from Sydney. "I'm going to make us some eggnog lattes," I announced amid my quest to orchestrate the perfect holiday moment. While enjoying them we admired the Christmas tree, laughing as my mischievous kittens, Bella and Leo, darted in and out of the pile of wrapped-and-beribboned gifts, bopping at the low-hanging baubles with their paws.

It was easy to love life when Dad came to town. He called me "Miss" and we talked about travel, books, and spirituality while sipping merlot. He was game to accompany me to any movie I wanted to see, and to foot the bill for yummy meals around town. From window-shopping on Rodeo Drive to sitting in the front row at *Jimmy Kimmel Live!*, we gladly posed as first-time tourists in the city I'd lived in for a decade. On this particular trip, we'd already plunged to the depths of Atlantis watching *Aquaman* in full glory on the gigantic IMAX screen at Universal Studios. We'd visited Abbot Kinney Boulevard for the best vegan pizza, sipped cocktails 71 floors above downtown L.A., and enjoyed fish and chips overlooking the ocean at Duke's in Malibu—Dad's favorite. After perusing the artworks at the Getty Center, we found ourselves grinning with childlike delight while holding our phones up to capture the spectacle of snowflakes falling from 60-degree skies over the Grove outdoor shopping mall. For someone who perpetually didn't "feel ready" to date, going out to restaurants, movies, and art galleries on those rare occasions when Dad was in town filled some kind of void, even if temporarily.

As was our tradition, I'd given Dad my Christmas wish list, so it was no surprise when I unboxed an Instant Pot, along with some gift cards to my favorite stores. Dad was impressed with his Duke's Malibu vintage surfboard T-shirt and the collection of new books I'd gifted him. As Leo jumped into the empty Instant Pot box, I looked down and noticed another gift beneath the tree. "This is for you, from Santa," Dad said. I picked up the gift with excited curiosity and, feeling its smooth, flat, square shape, deduced that it must be a hardcover recipe book. I smiled and peeled the wrapping paper off to reveal the front cover. There stood a tanned woman with long, flowing hair in a white bikini, gently leaning against a palm tree with the beach in the background. The cover of the book read: "*Flat Tummy Fast!* The Healthy Way to a Totally Toned Tummy in 14 Days." My smile faded as I crumpled in utter humiliation and pushed it away. "Ummm . . . thanks, Santa."

In his trying-to-help-but-not-doing-it-properly way, I know that Dad was expressing his concern about my well-being and trying to offer a solution. His not-so-subtle hints had been glaringly obvious lately! A few days prior we'd been driving down Pacific Coast Highway to Malibu Country Mart for smoothie bowls when I pointed up into the mountains surrounding Temescal Canyon and told him, "That's where I like to go hiking sometimes." In a deadpan tone he'd replied, "You haven't been there in a while, have you?"

Oh, the spontaneous joys of the unfiltered older generation. The truth was, I hadn't. Life had gotten in the way and somehow I'd gained 30 pounds since I'd last seen him, due to the stress of—I don't know what exactly, but it felt like a never-ending churn of hustle followed by exhaustion. I hadn't made time to exercise, and a recent scan had revealed an enlarged thyroid, indicating a thyroid hormone imbalance, which was contributing to my weight gain and fatigue. My confidence had taken a dive, so I wasn't dating or getting out much. I'd tried easing myself back into a regular exercise routine by attempting a 30-day exercise challenge, but when I missed Day 8, I felt like a failure and dropped out not long after. I was reaching for matcha lattes, sweet treats, or coffee to boost my energy. This worked for short periods of time, but then I would inevitably feel fatigued again. In the struggle to keep pace with today's reality, I lost sight of the dreams that once lit me up.

As someone watching her 30s slowly slipping away, I'd felt rising pressure to settle down. I hadn't meant to miss out on all the fun of marriage and kids; it just hadn't happened for me yet. I'd certainly been in love before and taken on the role of dutiful girlfriend, cooking my boyfriends elaborate dinners and arranging fun dates. After a couple of years of auditioning for the role of wifey, it had crushed my heart when each man had drifted away or told me he didn't see himself being "ready for marriage for another 10 years." I became disillusioned with love, raised my standards to a level that no person could live up to, and eventually lost any motivation to date at all. I secretly wasn't even sure that I was a good enough candidate as wife material. After a while it felt like everyone else had coupled up except for me. I'd resigned myself to having officially missed the boat on marriage.

My busy nine-to-five job at a nonprofit was fulfilling, but I'd always wanted to develop a side business where I could channel my creativity, offer value, and pay off the $10,000 debt that always seemed to linger. I would work to pay it off, and then more debt would accumulate. I struggled to identify a venture that would engage my creativity while serving a higher purpose, so I took on a lot of low-paying side hustles. On any given weeknight or weekend you could find me transcribing videos, selling items online, coordinating social media posts, planning events, and basically promoting everyone else's business while tying up all my free time. I was also prone to taking on additional projects at work to reinforce my value and winding up overwhelmed because I didn't want to fail or ask for help. When I wasn't hustling and exerting energy trying to control outcomes and create an air of perfection, I was recovering on the sofa watching Netflix and eating Häagen-Dazs ice cream. It felt like nothing I did created significant traction in improving my life.

In truth, my desires and goals weren't clearly defined. I sensed a vague, faraway vision of what I wanted stirring deep in my soul, but I didn't have a firm plan for how to get it. My growing desire was to protect myself and find stability by avoiding change at all costs! I frequently bowed out of meetups with friends and began to feel isolated. I knew I was meant for more, but didn't know how to make it happen.

On my birthday, a couple of my dearest friends invited me over for lunch to celebrate. The vibe was high tea in Paris, and they'd set up a cute tablescape with rose petals, elegant teacups, and Eiffel Tower napkins. It all felt really special, so I was taken aback when no sooner had the cake been brought out than one of my friends gave me a "talking to" about my life. She scolded me for not putting any effort into dating, improving my health, or moving my life in the direction of the things I truly wanted and deserved. Her words cut like the cake knife adorned with pink ribbon. I knew she was right, and I also knew how deeply she cared. Tears fell into my gluten-free chocolate chip birthday cake as the burning truth revealed itself. Why did her words hurt so much? Because they rang so true. Deep down, I didn't feel as though I'd accomplished the things in life that I truly wanted to.

Manifesting with Ease

Prompted by the recent series of truth bombs, that New Year's Eve I decided to transform my life by taking a mind-body-soul approach to manifesting my dreams. Rather than struggling to force outcomes, I wanted to align with my natural energy cycles to create the kind of lifestyle that would elevate my health, wealth, happiness, and love. I designed an energy-centric system to help me attract and align with my dreams, and I experienced positive results in each month that followed.

Part of my vision for my future self was to be a healthy, confident, loved-up woman, so a couple of months after I began tracking my energy cycles I invested in a gym membership. I chose a gym where I felt comfortable and inspired to transform my neglected, pushed-to-the-limit body back to her healthy self. I swayed, stretched, and strengthened my limbs in the lush, wood-paneled yoga space and revisited my clubbing nights in the mood-lit cycling studio, rocking in unison on spinning bikes to electronic dance music and motivational cheers from upbeat trainer Jilly. This became my happy place. I was leveraging my natural energy to fuel my workouts and choosing classes that aligned with each phase of my cycle. It wasn't long before I booked six sessions with a personal trainer.

Early one morning as I looked in the bathroom mirror to wash my face, I marveled at the thought of heading out to a 7:30 A.M. barre class. "Who is this person?" I smiled in disbelief and delight. The old me would never have entertained such a ridiculous idea. Paying attention to my body and treating it with care began to pay off in ways I couldn't have imagined. Aside from the sense that I was doing something deeply healing, I felt my body becoming stronger, and I had more energy to fire up my life and keep it in motion. I stopped hiding under loose, dark clothing and began expressing myself with happy colors and fun styles that aligned with my spirit. A new version of me was emerging, and as my confidence and happiness grew, I was also warming up to the idea of dating.

Although I'd felt like giving up on marriage in recent years, in my heart it was something I truly wanted. I'd always imagined myself being married someday, and since I was no longer subscribing to the "someday" syndrome, I knew it was time to start putting energy toward manifesting this desire. The thought of getting back into the dating pool after a few years of being single felt scary, but I decided to sign up for online dating and make plans to get out more to socialize. I attended evening classes, events, and mixers; volunteered in my spiritual community; hosted dinner parties; visited new places; and explored locations I was drawn to on weekends. I put feminine energy insights into practice and started having fun meeting potential matches.

Just as my dating life began to heat up, I was also experiencing positive results from moving my body regularly at the gym. I'd lost almost all of the 30 pounds of extra weight I'd been carrying around. As our sixth and final session came to an end, my personal trainer told me that my transformation had been one of the fastest he'd ever seen, and that he was quite amazed. He kept checking my records and adjusting the scale to be sure of what he was seeing. He congratulated me on "all the hard work and effort" I'd been putting in. As I drove home, I reflected on my progress. The truth was, it didn't feel as though I *had* put in any hard work or effort—it felt more like I'd been having fun and truly living in a way that brought me happiness.

I was living in alignment with my natural energy, and it was magnetizing my desires into reality—fast. I felt for the first time in years like I was doing what came naturally. Allowing myself joyful moments of play, resting when I felt like it, reaching out to friends when I was excited to connect, and spending time alone to reflect and plan when the mood struck. I felt happier and healthier than I had in a long time. I'd let go of struggle mode and feelings of lack. I started to say no to the things that just didn't light me up, and now wellness, love, happiness, and peace became my top priorities. I showed up on dates with high-vibe energy and started to spend most of my free time with one particular man.

Invest in Yourself

The decision to invest in a gym membership was one that I'd been putting off for years. What did it take to finally invest in myself? A health crisis. When it was no longer an option to shelve fitness in favor of stress, I made it work financially. I stopped buying junk food, downloading movies, going out for drinks, buying coffees and cakes, and picking up restaurant take-out meals—you know, all the fun stuff. Since learning the hard way that health truly is wealth, I made sure to prioritize eating nourishing whole foods, moving my body, and spending time outdoors to connect with nature. Investing in yourself doesn't have to cost a lot of money; lifestyle tweaks can be made to open up more opportunities for wellness. Prioritizing your well-being isn't selfish—it's essential. When you nurture your body with movement, fuel it with nourishing foods, and take intentional time to restore your mental and emotional balance, you create a ripple effect that enhances every area of your life. The returns on this investment are invaluable: greater resilience, improved focus, a deeper sense of purpose, and the vitality to pursue your dreams. Taking care of yourself equips you not only to thrive but also to serve those around you from a place of abundance. Investing in our wellness can feel like an unnecessary expense or indulgence, and yet we often allow ourselves to indulge in small, unhealthy "treats," trendy fast fashion, impulsive beauty buys, and knickknacks that just create more clutter. Dedicating time, energy, and resources to proper self-care can be accompanied by feelings of guilt, believing that those resources should go elsewhere.

This resistance can come at a cost. When we neglect our well-being, we risk burnout, diminished vitality, and a disconnect from our dreams and potential. We need to reframe self-investment as an act of empowerment and service—not just to ourselves but to others in our lives.

- - -

The holiday of July 4th soon came around, and I'd made plans to go to the Santa Monica beach with a girlfriend. We set up a little beach tent, laid out a picnic blanket, played some music, and started snacking on watermelon. There we were, having our fun girly moment, chatting about boys, sharing our latest adventures, taking selfies, sipping cold drinks, and enjoying the celebration as the warmth of the sun beamed down and the waves rolled in. I took a deep breath of fresh ocean air and soaked up the good-feeling vibes—and then it struck me. Here I was, feeling free, happy, and confident and enjoying the beach . . . while wearing a bikini! I laughed out loud as I remembered Santa's ever-so-thoughtful Christmas present of six months earlier, the *Flat Tummy Fast!* book. I'd almost forgotten about the incident—a memory that would have left me feeling down and insecure in the past. Speaking of Santa, I had e-mailed Dad a photo of me receiving a big bunch of long-stemmed red roses from the man I was dating. He replied, saying, "Well, Miss, I have never seen you looking so radiant."

Following natural energy cycles propelled me toward the future I had been dreaming of. If only I had known about the power of cycles earlier. I'd found a more aligned way to live than trying to fit myself into a daily schedule of energy. Magically, there was a time for everything. When the opportunity to work on fun events and projects came up, I had plenty of energy to take on those enjoyable side jobs that would help me pay off credit card debt. I started to invest time into learning about topics I was interested in, growing my knowledge, and following my curiosity. It wasn't long before I felt unshackled from any feelings of heaviness and healed from health issues, hormonal imbalance, and burnout. I was having a blast dating, paying off debt through work I loved, learning about topics that interested me, and finally being in charge of my energy. Not only did I feel excited about the future, I was also enjoying the present.

Decide. Then Take Aligned Action

We so often wait for permission from others to deviate from the well-journeyed path. This hesitation stems from an instinct to protect ourselves. When we consider acting in ways counter to the popular approach, it can bring up subconscious fears. For me, making the decision proved to be half the battle won. Coming out of my head and getting in touch with my body might not have aligned with the dictates of hustle culture, but it aligned with my goals to achieve my best health. Feeling borderline unhealthy and unfit for a long time had left me worn out and ready to try something dramatically different. Being open to finding love, despite the fears of not being ready and not feeling like I was enough, aligned with my soul's desire to share my life with someone. The desire to find a creative outlet that enabled me to share my gifts with the world and call in extra money felt scary but exciting. Conviction in decision-making paves the way for intentional actions that are in resonance with your heart and soul desires.

Misaligned

In looking back on my journey of breaking free from burnout, combined with the knowledge I've gained since by studying integrative nutrition, lifestyle medicine, and hormone health and by working with clients, I've discovered that there are energetic forces in life that can keep us stuck if we become entangled in them. The good news is that there are powerful forces we can align with—ones that can propel us toward living a life of wellness where we feel empowered to manifest our heart and soul desires into reality.

We are living in an age of evolutionary mismatch—a time when our environment has drastically changed, but our biology is still wired for the world of our ancestors. This is one of the driving forces causing our misalignment. Our genes, shaped by millions of years of evolution, are designed to respond to natural rhythms, nutrient-dense whole foods, physical activity, and relatively low levels of stress. Today, we lead sedentary lifestyles, and we're surrounded by processed foods, artificial light, and a constant barrage of stressors. This disconnect between our genetic programming and the modern environment creates a state of misalignment that can result in negative effects on our wellness such as chronic disease, hormonal dysregulation, mental health challenges, and more.

But there's hope: By aligning with our natural energy cycles and implementing small shifts that work in our favor, we can change direction. Thanks to epigenetics, we hold remarkable power to influence our bodies, even at the genetic level. Our genes are not static, they're responsive to their environment. Aging doesn't have to be defined by decline or disease. Instead, we have the potential to thrive. We are being called to take greater sovereignty over our choices, even if it means going against the norm and embracing a path less traveled.

Rewriting Your Story with Epigenetics

Epigenetics is the study of how lifestyle factors like diet, sleep, stress, and even exposure to toxins can switch genes on or off without altering the underlying DNA sequence. These gene expressions are our body's way of trying to adapt to external triggers. An example of epigenetics in action is the effect of cruciferous vegetables that are rich in sulforaphane (such as broccoli and kale) on gene expression. Sulforaphane activates the Nrf2 pathway, a key regulator of antioxidant and detoxification genes, helping the body neutralize free radicals, reduce inflammation, and support cellular health.[1] Consuming cruciferous vegetables can "switch on" beneficial genes, promoting a healthier internal environment and potentially reducing the risk of developing chronic diseases. Our choices hold incredible power, and we now know play a more significant role than ever in shaping our wellness. By making intentional choices—like eating nourishing foods, reducing stress, and engaging in regular movement—we can influence gene expression in ways that support our longevity and align us with the vibrant life we envision. Just as our genes can be reprogrammed, so too can we rewrite our destinies.

Feminine wisdom has been suppressed for centuries, yet when we reconnect with our body, and the natural rhythms of the moon and seasons, we can tap into the momentum of natural energies as if it were second nature. To truly thrive and magnetize our dreams into manifestation, we must break free of the forces that keep us sleepwalking through life. If we're not aligning with natural energy cycles to manage our energy and create meaningful change, we risk being pulled under by external forces and energies that don't serve us. Now is the time to identify what's been holding us back from manifesting our dream lives.

What follows are 10 signs that you may be feeling misaligned with the beneficial energies of natural cycles as you try to cope with difficult modern-day phenomena and conditions that have become so common, we've come to accept them as part of "normal" life. I've experienced these forces of misalignment myself over the years. It's time to break free from these energetic constraints and begin aligning with our own powerful energy cycles. The first step is to identify where you might be misaligned. Pay attention to these 10 signs and how they may be affecting you, and know that there is a way to release these patterns and begin to thrive!

If you are experiencing one or more of the following, you may be feeling misaligned:

- **Meant for More.** Do you ever feel like life is just okay and that deep down, you long for something more? You're going through the motions, busy with daily demands, but a quiet voice within whispers that you're meant for greater things. You long for a purpose and sense that your current path isn't fully aligned with your soul's desires. This can cause you to feel unfulfilled, or unsure of how to bridge the gap between your current reality and where you want to be. The life you truly crave feels just out of reach, pushed further and further away by urgent demands. Perhaps you're not even sure what your true heart and soul desires really are? You catch glimpses of a greater vision, giving you moments of clarity, but they slip away, buried under a pile of to-dos. Your yearning for more isn't just dissatisfaction—it's your soul calling for alignment, for a life that lights you up, brings your dreams to life, and positively impacts others. It's a clue that there's more waiting for you—a deeper level of fulfillment, a truer purpose. Listen to that voice. It knows the way.

- **Information Overload.** Another screenshot, another statistic, another word of advice from a friend—but confusion persists and it remains difficult to fully commit to a decision or create lasting change. Hours spent mulling over conflicting information can leave you feeling stuck and frustrated (ever tried googling "what's the healthiest diet"?). In an attempt to get a handle on things, you collect and categorize data. Checklists, saved posts, pinned recipes, articles, cheat sheets, fitness routines—all are amassed in digital folders that rarely get revisited. With every false start, failed attempt, or shortfall in completing those ambitious 30-day challenges (which seemed like a good idea when you started), you lose trust in your abilities. Self-doubt and the noise of external stimuli can drown out the whispers of inner wisdom. Decision fatigue makes it difficult to launch plans into action. After weighing every option, you convince yourself it's simply not the right time to pursue your dreams or embark upon something new. Mind chatter dominates, making it difficult to switch off and contributing to brain fog and troubled sleep. Late-night problem-solving becomes overwhelming as mental exhaustion eventually kicks in. Cutting through the static and aligning with a clear pathway to meaningful growth will entail some soul-searching and sharpening of your intuition. Are you ready to press pause on all the noise and hone the skills needed to turn your dreams into reality?

- **Struggle Mode.** An idyllic vacation spot with white-sand beaches graces your screen, but it's quickly being obscured by an array of files and folders. There's work to be done, after all, and not many are up to the task or can be trusted to do it properly—except for you. Prone to perfectionism, you take control and may even be accused of micromanaging at times. You dream of a day at the spa, but fear what might happen if you dare to take your hands off the wheel. The passions that light you up are pushed off to "someday" in the future. But that day isn't today—there are problems that need fixing. Even in the face of challenges, you strive for stability and success by dedicating your time, energy, and resources, yet the compensation or recognition received rarely matches the effort you expend. The daily grind can feel like treading water—working hard to barely keep up with expenses, leading to exhaustion. It becomes impossible to tap into a sense of gratitude or peacefulness when your inner critic reminds you that you're "just not doing enough." In relationships, you're often the one keeping the connection alive, which can feel like a burden when your efforts go unmatched. When life starts to go smoothly, it can feel almost too good to be true, leaving you anxious and anticipating where things might unravel. Lucky breaks seem to happen to others, and they make it look effortless. But what if luck has nothing to do with it? What if the secret to success lies in mastering the balancing of both stability and flow? You've already mastered the ability to remain focused, disciplined, and resilient, creating a stable foundation for growth. Now, it's time to explore your capacity to flow with creativity, tap into your intuition, embrace change, and cultivate trust in the Universe by aligning with the natural rhythms of life and leveraging their energies to your advantage! Harmonizing the forces of stability and flow creates a life that feels both secure *and* inspired, empowering you to truly thrive.

- **Against the Clock.** It's 3 P.M. and you're deep in an energy slump. The caffeine kick from your morning latte has long worn off and you're craving a sugary pick-me-up to power you through the last stretch of your looming project deadline. Working late would mean missing your fitness class, which is at the very top of your "non-negotiable" list of daily routines. Having to skip a daily habit leaves you feeling guilty, or even wanting to give up altogether. Life often feels like a race that can't be won—you're constantly chasing time, striving to finish one thing before the next begins. This can compel you to feel reactive, detached, or unmoored. It's tough to justify stepping away for too long, so when you do take a break, it's hard to truly relax, so you often end up doing something productive instead. Watching your peers advance in their careers and achieve personal milestones can leave you feeling left behind as you compare your progress to theirs. The perpetual pressure to meet daily demands and gain a competitive edge at work can drive you to seek short cuts or quick fixes in other areas of life instead of taking time to address underlying causes of imbalance. Amid the rush of activity it's easy to overlook opportunities to implement sustainable practices for lasting change. Time waits for no man, as the saying goes, but the relentless 24-hour clock is an unforgiving structure that doesn't align with the natural rhythms of a woman. Imagine making a shift to a more spacious paradigm where *energy* is queen—setting you free to breathe, recharge, catch a sunset or two, and still achieve your goals.

- **Lacking Confidence.** "Hey, I love how the color of your sweater really matches your eyes—you look so pretty," compliments a colleague. "Oh gosh, this thing?" you reply. "I got it at a discount store. Ughh, I feel tired today, so I probably look sleepy. You look great, though! I love your dress!" Why does it always feel so awkward to be given a compliment? It's like being in the spotlight when you'd prefer not to draw attention to yourself. Sometimes small insecurities have a way of multiplying. Imagine this scenario—you're up for a promotion at work and the new role will require you to regularly give presentations to the board. You visualize giving engaging pitches and updates about innovative projects that will take the organization to the next level. Plus a promotion would also enable you to upgrade your apartment and move to a better part of town. Then a familiar voice chimes in: "Know your limits. You'll never be good at speaking in front of an audience. Remember that time you failed? You'll look like an idiot!" And so you play it small by not allowing yourself to shine and perform well at the interviews. Learning that you didn't get the promotion initially brings a wave of relief, but it soon turns to disappointment over having missed a big opportunity. Deflecting compliments, dimming your light, and engaging in negative self-talk are signs that you may secretly believe you're undeserving of your desires or that you must earn them by meeting impossibly high standards. You may fear expressing your authentic self, voicing your opinions, revealing your spiritual side, or showing up online, worried you'll be seen as "not enough" even though you have valuable insights to share. This mindset can result in self-sabotage, procrastination, or the inability to fully own your success. Energetically, it can also repel the things you actually want to receive in life. Confidence grows by taking small, consistent steps toward self-empowerment, celebrating your progress, and recognizing your inherent worth. Practicing receiving something as simple as a compliment prepares you to graciously receive your manifestations, unlocking greater fulfillment and success.

- **Isolation.** Life can give us so many reasons to retreat. We may find ourselves declining a series of invitations from friends or family to take time to heal our body, heart, or soul. Eventually, hiding from life becomes all too comfortable. Not interacting or socializing as we used to can make it that much harder to connect again. What leads us to retreat? Maybe we feel misunderstood, fatigued, or weighed down by past traumas or emotions. It could be an urge for hyper-independence to prove to ourselves that we'll be "just fine" alone. We may be surrounded by people, yet keep our true self under wraps. Taking space for yourself is a good thing, especially if you're a sensitive person, an empath, or someone who needs quiet time to reflect and process. But humans are also wired for connection with others, as it provides us with the necessities of love, acceptance, and a sense of security. These social bonds are important for our well-being, fulfilling emotional and psychological needs. Feelings of doubt and fear about the future can be overwhelming, but by embracing the natural ebb and flow of life, we can move beyond these limitations. Movement and change are essential elements of growth, and if trying something new doesn't turn out as expected, you can always pivot to something else. Life operates in cycles, with a new season always on the horizon. Embrace the flow and let these natural cycles of energy uplift you. You'll find that you're never alone in this journey of co-creation.

- **Going with the Crowd.** Do you ever find yourself looking for external validation or seeking permission before making a decision? When we put too much weight on the opinions of those around us, it becomes harder to hear the quiet voice within ourselves. Although it might seem easier in the moment, suppressing your needs and desires to fit in with the expectations of others can leave you feeling disconnected from your authentic self. Without establishing your own clearly defined path, you risk becoming part of someone else's agenda or getting swept up in trends that don't align with your unique vision. Have you ever caught yourself being overly agreeable or changing course to meet someone else's demands, all the while wishing you had the courage and freedom to follow your own path? Staying silent to maintain peace doesn't foster growth, or allow for authentic connection. You may also secretly worry about what your parents, your ex, or Jenny from high school might think if you do what you *really* want to do. Learning to trust your inner guidance so you can stand firm in your choices and embrace your sovereignty will help you find liberation and empowerment. While connecting with others is important, it's just as important to honor your own truths. By aligning your actions with your heart and soul desires, you can create a life that reflects your true self.

- **Not Embodied.** When we're not embodied, we're living mostly in our heads—overflowing with ideas, insights, and inspiration—while our body's signals and needs fade quietly into the background. Have you ever felt like your body can't keep up with your mind? Do you tend to prioritize mental tasks when life gets stressful? You may barely notice your scrunched posture, shallow breathing, or muscle stiffness. Before you know it, months have whizzed by without you having shown yourself any body love by moving; gently stretching; allowing physical touch; nourishing your skin; working muscles; taking deep, cleansing breaths; or shaking the tension out of your arms and legs. When you override your body's needs for too long, it can feel like a stranger. Another clue that we're not fully embodied is when our knowledge hasn't yet shaped our habits. Do you study something endlessly, yet never fully live it? Maybe you light up when the topic of conversation turns to nutrition because you're eager to share your knowledge with a group of friends. You excitedly present the newest scientific findings and recipes you've collected to convince them of the benefits of a new diet and fitness plan that you're enthralled by. "This sounds great; how did it work out for you?" one of them asks. You squirm a little as you explain that you haven't tried it yet, but you want to start soon. The truth is, you've been mentally stalking everything about this new regimen for months but haven't actually put any of it into practice. Your knowledge is boundless—imagine how empowered you would feel if even a small portion of your intellectual treasures could make it into embodiment. Your body is an integral member of the mind-body-soul trio, and all of them are important for manifesting. Embodiment is where change happens. To bypass the body is to avoid real and lasting change. Try checking in with her and asking her how she feels today and what she needs.

- **Escapism.** Sometimes it's just easier to drop issues into the "too hard" basket and move on to more comforting or pleasurable pursuits. Heartbreak, feeling let down by your bestie, getting critical feedback from a colleague, losing a loved one, job, or pet—life can feel pretty terrible at times. Perhaps you're tired of being weighed down by gloom, stress, or oversize emotional baggage and wish it would all just evaporate. Sure, you've considered working through your troubles, maybe through journaling, self-reflection, mind-body therapies, emotional release, or an honest conversation or two. But instead, you prefer to just skip straight to the part where you already feel healed, liberated, and blissful! This impulse could cause you to jump from one activity to another, chasing instant satisfaction. Bingeing on junk food and reality shows until 3 A.M., shopping online until your credit card nears its limit, overindulging in wine or other substances, obsessing over a new crush every month, or driving around town all day in search of the best mochi doughnut—over time, the anticipation of something bringing happiness can outweigh the actual experience of it, leaving you constantly chasing that fleeting high. Ongoing patterns of excessive, obsessive, rebellious, or risky behaviors may temporarily drown out troubles, but they also come with unwanted side effects and can be difficult to quit. But maybe living for the moment isn't delivering the lasting results your soul truly craves in your search for vibrant health, satisfying relationships, peace of mind, confidence, prosperity, self-acceptance.

Your natural zest for life, creativity, and imagination are powerful forces that can magnetize your dreams toward you. A little self-reflection and inner work will help you clear out emotional debris and clarify your heart and soul desires. By aligning with the supportive structure of natural cycles, you can direct your energy toward designing a life that loves you back.

- **Distraction.** You'd be crushing your goals and soaring toward success right now if only life didn't keep getting in the way of your dreams. There are just so many things vying for your attention that it's no wonder you have FOMO. Constant notifications, flash sales, viral trends, DMs on multiple platforms, subscriptions, and pop-ups all cause scattered, reactive energy. You may be prone to distraction, but your intentions are golden. It generally starts out as an earnest endeavor to explore a new field of study, find methods to enhance your ability to form habits, or figure out ways to make extra cash on the side. Somewhere along the way you find yourself watching a family from Ohio renovate a cottage in the French countryside. Have you ever been on the verge of launching a passion project, only to have an opportunity to take on extra work you don't enjoy pop up? The money is less than your usual rate, but it's hard to turn down any financial offer, even though it pulls you further away from your dream venture. Or how about sidelining your health and wellness goals in favor of happy hour, window-shopping, endless tasks, or watching TV? Your friends know they can count on you when they need to hash out a plan to get their ex back, lament an office drama, or theorize on how to escape the city in the event of a zombie apocalypse. While it's natural to want to support friends, family members, and co-workers, becoming too entangled in OPD (other people's drama) can lead to burnout, a lack of personal focus, and neglect of your own well-being—like staying up late to listen to a friend complain about trivial things instead of getting a good night's sleep. If it feels like your goals and dreams have been slipping away with each passing day, month, and year, then it's time to play catch-up. Transforming desires into tangible results can feel daunting. What if you could bypass the traditional linear pathway of laboring, hustling, and proving and instead use intention, passion, and energetic alignment to help you collapse time and create big shifts? Don't allow life's distractions to interrupt you in living out *your* unique storyline—is it an adventure? A romance? A tale of success? Or one of strength and healing? Focus on the plot that lights you up the most and pursue it with a healthy dose of main-character energy.

If you're nodding, raising your hand, or announcing "*I feel seen!*" about any of these (or even parts of them), know that I've been there too and have experienced all of these energetic influences at one time or another. In fact, these forces of misalignment are considered a normal part of life by many. However, when we are living in alignment with our heart and soul desires and utilizing the natural energies available to help us manifest our dreams, these ways of being are fleeting moments at best and definitely not the norm.

Getting stuck in misaligned forces could cost you time that could otherwise be devoted to personal growth, well-being, revealing your purpose, and achieving your fullest potential. In subtle or powerful ways, they can usher you down a path that saps your energy and limits your ability to flourish. They do this by using the power of momentum. The good news is that momentum works both ways. While it can lead us down a path that doesn't serve us, changing direction allows each positive step toward our dreams and goals to build upon the last, creating a cumulative force that gains speed and power over time.

Momentum and Manifesting

Momentum in physics is defined as mass multiplied by velocity. The greater the mass and velocity, the more momentum something has, making it harder to stop it or change its direction.

Manifesting involves a similar dynamic. The "mass" represents the feelings tied to what we wish to manifest, while the "velocity" reflects our energetic alignment over time. When we want to manifest something, it's ultimately the emotions those manifestations evoke that we seek. By consistently aligning ourselves with natural energies to move us closer to our desired feelings, we strengthen the momentum of our manifestations while exerting less effort. We can become better manifesters by drawing inspiration from the natural rhythms and momentum inherent in nature and the Universe.

As the moon moves through space, it maintains its momentum due to the gravitational pull of the Earth, which keeps it in orbit. It would take a huge force to stop or redirect the momentum of the moon because it's energetically and magnetically attached to a larger environment—the Earth. In the same way, we can anchor ourselves to environments that contribute to our momentum toward the things we wish to manifest. There are places and spaces that can help us naturally align with our desired feelings and dreams. For example, if your dream is to write a blog, you'll want to create a cozy nook at home that's conducive to writing, or to frequent a quiet café or library where you can settle in to craft your blog posts. If you wish to manifest a stronger body by working out more, you might want to choose the gym that makes you feel comfortable, uplifted, and inspired instead of the closest affordable gym in your location. Align with the environment that makes you feel as though you are already a writer or someone who enjoys working out regularly.

Have you ever noticed that migrating birds fly in a V formation? They leverage aerodynamic principles to conserve energy and maintain momentum. The lead bird creates a slipstream, allowing the birds behind it to glide with less effort. When the lead bird gets tired, another bird takes its place. This cooperative behavior not only saves energy, but also ensures that the flock maintains speed over long distances. Studies have shown that birds in a V formation can increase their distance by up to 70 percent compared to flying alone.[2] The birds take advantage of the updraft created by the flapping of the wings of the bird ahead, allowing them to glide and maintain altitude with less effort. By following the paths of those who have achieved what you desire and getting involved in supportive communities, you can remove any distance or friction between you and your desired manifestation and tap into the power of momentum to propel yourself forward. A practical example of this would be joining a female entrepreneur network if you are starting a business. This may sound like just another commitment you don't have time for, but the people you meet there will have already traversed the pathways you are about to travel and can offer you priceless advice and connections that enable you to take the kinds of shortcuts you never could have imagined just by being part of their cooperative network.

We can't talk about momentum without bringing up the classic example of a snowball rolling downhill. The snowball effect is a powerful metaphor for understanding momentum, especially in the context of manifestation. Just as a small snowball rolling down a hill accumulates more snow and gains speed, when we take small positive actions toward our goals and manifestations (such as our Cycle Habits—more on that later), it becomes easier and easier to begin living in alignment with a more elevated vibration. Eventually, the momentum becomes so powerful that it propels you toward achieving your goals with greater ease. This doesn't just work with actions; it can work with mindset as well. Your thoughts and emotions continue to influence your reality at all times. If we feel misaligned, we can make it a practice to stop focusing on the thoughts that bring us fears and doubts and instead notice small things to appreciate. Start collecting these positive things by writing them down each day. Where our attention goes, our energy flows. If we do this consistently, our positive expectations and thoughts can build momentum over time, leading to significant changes in our lives. Start with small steps and build from there. Just take the first step. Immerse yourself in good emotions regularly and acknowledge the micro-manifestations that occur in daily life. Cultivate an attitude of gratitude for small wins, and keep it rolling.

The key to using momentum for manifesting is consistency, and the key for making it all effortless is to align with natural energies and cycles already available all around you in life, the Universe, and your body. By practicing the Cycle Magic method to manifest your dreams, you're working *with* nature's energy rather than against it.

How Does It Feel to Be Aligned?

So you might be wondering . . . having aligned myself with natural energy cycles, where has this momentum taken me? Have I been able to manifest my truest desires by leveraging powerful, supportive energies? By way of an update, I'm happy to report that kitties Bella and Leo now have a cat daddy who loves them just as much as I do. We met four months into my manifesting journey, and I became engaged on Christmas Eve of that year. Tying the knot in front of friends and family in a chapel by the ocean was an experience I'll always remember. I have a wonderful new family whom I love dearly and look forward to spending time with. We live a short distance from the beach and are surrounded by hiking trails, lakes, and beautiful coastal resorts.

Following my deep desire for healthy living and wellness, I've gained certifications in the areas of integrative nutrition and hormone health as well as lifestyle medicine approaches taught at Harvard Medical School. My passion for spirituality and universal energies led me to deepen my studies in those areas and become a Moonologer and Law of Attraction practitioner. I now help women recover from burnout, rebalance their hormones, and attract their heart and soul desires into manifestation. I'm showing up in my career with more intention and a higher vibe and working on dream projects that fill me with a sense of purpose. I attend inspiring events and meet incredible entrepreneurial women, all while taking plenty of time to rest, get a good night's sleep, visit the spa once a month, and incorporate luscious self-care habits into my life that help me feel rejuvenated and confident.

I was perpetually in and out of debt and knew very little about the status of my 401(k), but I now have a self-managed investment portfolio with more than a year's worth of living expenses saved, and I very much enjoy researching stocks, growing my dividend income, and trading options. (Yes, even the stock market works in cycles!)

After clinging to my reliable but outdated Prius for over a decade I decided it was time to manifest my dream car. I began using Cycle Magic visualization and embodiment techniques to help make my self-driving Telsa Model Y dream a reality. I call her Spirit, and she makes it so much easier for me to conserve my energy while getting where I need to go safely and with *way* less stress and effort.

It brings me joy to follow my intuitive and creative nudges—whether it's painting artwork for my office, designing a fitness closet, or coming up with new recipes for The Cycle Diet collection using brightly colored seasonal produce that nourishes me and my clients through every phase of the cycle.

Someday **Begins Now**

For years, I was unknowingly stuck in the grip of energetic forces that held me back. I had visions of the life I deeply desired, but it always felt just out of reach. I believed the things I wanted would take years to achieve, so I often procrastinated. Failed attempts to force things into existence or stick to daily habits left me feeling unworthy of achieving them. A life of wellness, a loving relationship, time to rest and reconnect with nature, abundant resources, and the ability to follow my joy and curiosity to create a meaningful venture and share transformative ideas with others—these dreams remained tucked away, waiting for a *someday* that never seemed to arrive. But the belief that we have no time to pursue our desires or that it will take years for them to manifest is an illusion. I discovered that I could start leveraging natural rhythms and cycles to propel me forward right away. My desires are no longer shelved for a future version of myself to enjoy. I bend time by living my dream life today, so it begins to unfold before my eyes in record time—because I'm no longer measuring time, I'm measuring energy.

Most important is that I have manifested peace of mind and trust, allowing me to make decisions without being reactive or emotionally triggered. I've replaced a mindset of lack with a spirit of abundance. Letting go of comparisons has helped me focus on the things in my life that bring me authentic happiness. I no longer chase the illusion that "the grass is greener" elsewhere, nor do I dwell in victim consciousness or self-sabotage.

As an empath, I once internalized others' judgments and saw myself through their eyes instead of truly knowing my authentic self. Now, I've built the courage to branch out, make my mark, and cultivate confidence. I rely less on the opinions of others and more on my own inner knowing and my alignment with the force of creation. I no longer feel like I'm facing life's challenges alone. I feel guided, and notice signs and signals all around me. Synchronicities—winks from the Universe—have become a natural part of my life. It feels like I've unlocked my superpowers and receive the right information at the right time and have the resources I need show up just when I need them to invest in my journey.

I now measure success by the peace I feel within, and by having the ability to co-create a life that brings me both joy and purpose. Each day, I take time to appreciate what I have. I've released the urge to control, and plan every outcome. Life unfolds pretty effortlessly moment by moment. My approach to life is completely transformed. I now co-create it with powerful energies—ones that support, guide, and inspire me every step of the way.

Where I once experienced fear, lack, and uncertainty about where life might take me, I now have an inner knowing of where I'm headed. I might not see the big picture, but I trust in each divinely inspired step along the way as I look back in awe at what has unfolded so far. As long as I continue to co-create with universal energies and cycles for the purpose of expansion instead of trying to swim against the energetic tide or do battle alone, I know I'll be moving in the right direction.

I've been in your shoes. I've read inspirational self-improvement books and thought to myself, *That's okay for her—she had support, or a mentor, or money.* There was always a reason I allowed others to live fully while convincing myself it wasn't possible for me. But I want you to know this: If I could change the direction of my life, anyone can. Even if you feel like your dreams are slipping away, time is running out, you're not the right candidate, or you've tried and failed before—whatever the story that you're telling yourself is—focus on even the smallest opening of possibility. That tiny opening is all you need because change is possible, and it can happen for you. It might feel like other people have discovered the magic formula or mindset to manifest what they want, but you're still searching. Everything you need is available to you. The Cycle Magic journey offers more than 70 practices aligned with powerful, natural energy cycles and rhythms. This energy doesn't favor anyone—it's here for all of us. And it's ready for you!

This is where I hold your hands and tell you that we're going to explore these exiting manifesting practices together right here! And then we both scream "Eeeeeeeeek!" and jump up and down with excitement. Metaphorically, of course.

Chapter 2

CYCLE BASICS

• • • • • • • •

Once you've followed every trail, tested every door, and pressed against every edge; once you've willed, compelled, and still fallen short, look beyond, look within, and recalibrate.

Manage Your Energy, Not Your Time

What if, instead of trying to squeeze more tasks onto your daily to-do list, you tuned in to something deeper—your energy? Imagine knowing exactly when your energy is at its peak and aligning your most important activities with those moments. Time is finite, but energy is dynamic—it ebbs and flows through the day, the month, and even the seasons. It can influence everything from how you feel emotionally to what's happening physically in your body. Too often, we work against natural energies, leaving ourselves drained and frustrated. But shifting from managing your time to managing your energy lets you tap into something powerful.

Aligning with my natural cycles of energy unlocked innate wisdom within me, and it superseded the need to micromanage my time. I let go of perfection and surrendered to the natural phases of both restful and action-oriented energies. My body had revealed a powerful wisdom that was now activated and unleashed into my life. Everyday tasks that had kept me stuck and under the illusion of being "busy" began to flow with less effort and more ease. I used my energy intentionally and began to enjoy being immersed in an activity and being in the moment. This is known as the *flow state*.[1] I had learned as a spiritual concept and a scientific theory that everything is made up of energy. Now I had firsthand experience of this at work in my life. Everything is energy, and it moves in cycles. By learning to honor my energy, I discovered a way to live and work that felt deeply aligned and far less exhausting.

It's time to stop swimming against the stream and align with a greater force of energy to help attract and manifest your desires. This isn't about a huge, dramatic shift. It's about small, intentional changes. It's about trusting your natural rhythms, aligning with the energy already surrounding you, and letting it guide you toward what you desire. Life will become less about effort and more about alignment—and more joyful and deeply satisfying.

Rediscover Your Feminine Energy

As feminine energy beings living within a masculine structure of time and productivity, it's no wonder we often feel misaligned, overwhelmed, or disconnected from our natural rhythms. The constant push for linear progress and external achievement doesn't always honor the cyclical, intuitive nature of feminine energy.

Female hormones ebb and flow on a near-monthly cycle, with our energy-boosting hormones fluctuating through four distinct phases: menstrual, follicular, ovulatory, and luteal. These hormonal shifts influence everything from our energy level to our mood, creativity, and focus. What feels like a productive day in one phase may not feel the same in another. In contrast, men experience potent secretions of the "can-do" hormone testosterone in a steady and reliable pattern throughout the day, with levels significantly higher than those found in women.[2]

The moon cycle is a powerful expression of natural feminine rhythms, especially for women who don't experience a regular menstrual cycle. The moon's phases tap into different energies throughout the month: The new moon encourages rest and setting intentions, the full moon boosts confident embodiment, and the waning and waxing phases promote personal growth.

By aligning with these feminine cycles, we can enhance our intuition and balance the flow between action and rest. Embracing windows of restfulness during part of our cycle creates space to tap into the more metaphysical gifts that come with the feminine. We can strike a balance between being in our feminine energy (which is creative, intuitive, nonlinear) and utilizing our masculine energy (best for planning, initiating, structuring) to help us shape our ideas into reality. Rest sounds like a passive pursuit, but it can be very empowering. It can provide shortcuts through intuitive insights that are heard only when we journey into the stillness. We may receive a nudge to visit a certain friend, or to go to a particular place, or to explore a specific topic, and the next thing we know, it opens up a new possibility for enhancing our health, prosperity, relationships, or happiness—those things we truly desire in life.

What is true empowerment for women? It's not about trying to control every aspect of life. When we push our body too far into the stress zone, cortisol rises and no diet, workout routine, or juice cleanse will cause the change we desire if we consistently exist in fight-or-flight. True empowerment is having the ability to create enough space in your life to rest when your body needs it, to reflect upon and process emotions and events, to receive energetic cues for shifting into action mode, and to take time to enjoy and celebrate life. The Cycle Magic system creates the structure necessary for your feminine essence to thrive.

> Regardless of gender, if you consider yourself a feminine energy being or you're somebody who wants to be more in touch with their feminine energy, the Cycle Magic system is here to assist you in connecting with the deeply healing cycles and rhythms of the feminine. You'll discover practices that invite you into a state of "being" as a reprieve from the masculine "doing" energies so you can reconnect with your superpowers of intuition, creativity, and manifesting magic.

Manifesting Your Desires

The Law of Attraction asserts that "like attracts like" and everything in the Universe operates at a certain frequency or vibration. By raising your own frequency—by cultivating positive thoughts, emotions, and actions—you align yourself with higher vibrational experiences and attract what you desire. This is an essential component of the process of manifesting, but it's not the whole story. How do we maintain a higher vibration? Is it even realistic? How do we clear out the static that leads to self-sabotage when life feels too good to be true? How do we tell if our desires come from a selfish place or a deeply aligned one?

Desiring things is in our nature. We all have desires, and everything you want is attached to the way it's going to make you feel. Even physical desires like houses, cars, and relationships are really energetic desires for feelings of safety, happiness, and love. The nature of desires is that they never end—they evolve and deepen as we grow. We're always manifesting, but many of us are doing it the hard way. Our thoughts, emotions, and actions constantly shape our reality. Whether we're intentional about it or not, the energy we put out attracts experiences, opportunities, and outcomes that align with it. Manifestation isn't just about big dreams—it's the everyday process of how our inner world creates our outer world. By becoming more conscious of this, we can shift from manifesting by default to manifesting with purpose.

There's an intuitive, revolutionary way to manifest your truest heart and soul desires—one that allows you to work with universal energies rather than against them. By embracing this holistic approach to manifesting, we can step into a flow that aligns with our deepest desires and highest potential. It's not about forcing outcomes, but about trusting the natural rhythms of the Universe and letting them guide us toward the life we're truly meant to live.

Selfish Season

Do you ever feel a twinge of guilt when you take time for self-care? This feeling of resistance kept my light dim for years—until I made the decision to tend to my wellness. It took me a matter of months to turn my life around. I achieved a better level of health and fitness, went from being single to being engaged, redirected my creative energy toward things that truly lit me up, learned to feel worthy enough to receive good things, and progressed substantially along the path of becoming debt-free. I had invested a few months of what might be considered "selfish" time, but in reality, every small change I made helped me feel better and better. I was able to show up in life with a higher vibration and feel more inspired and invigorated. I made time to connect and socialize with friends and family, create more value at my workplace, build new friendships, and give back to my community. Along the way, I learned to say no to certain things that, surprisingly, worked out just fine without my involvement. So, in hindsight, was this really a selfish time? Or did it just feel that way at the beginning because I wasn't accustomed to putting my focus on my growth? If you feel the need to focus on your well-being, I invite you to embrace your own "selfish season," even if just for a month, while you get started with the Cycle Magic system.

- -

When we become familiar with the energy cycles around us, we can work in alignment with them to manifest more easily and gracefully. It just feels good to the core. Life can seem unpredictable at times, but if we routinely align with supportive energies, we can face challenges with more resiliency. This builds our trust in the natural cycles of the Universe and our body. Natural energy cycles and rhythms are predictable and will always be there for us (even beyond our menstruating years), and we can tap into them at any moment.

Here are some of the energetic cycles and rhythms that you will learn to leverage during your Cycle Magic journey.

The Menstrual Cycle

Our menstrual cycle is a natural, energetic rhythm that profoundly impacts our physical, emotional, and mental well-being. A full cycle can range from 21 to 35 days, typically lasting about 28 days. As our hormones shift throughout the month, they influence everything from our energy level to our cravings and emotional needs. During the menstrual phase, energy tends to be lower, and it's a time for rest and reflection. As we move into the follicular phase, a rise in the hormone estrogen boosts energy and awakens creativity and motivation, making it an ideal time to initiate new projects. Ovulation brings a surge in confidence and connection, while the luteal phase may feel more introspective, with a heightened need for comfort and self-care thanks to the calming effects of the hormone progesterone. Honoring and aligning with these cycles can help reduce stress, restore balance, and support overall health, allowing us to feel more grounded, energized, and in tune with our bodies throughout the month.

The Moon Cycle

The moon cycle, much like the menstrual cycle, operates in powerful, energetic phases. A full cycle takes approximately 29 days. The moon has long been associated with feminine energy, symbolizing intuition, emotions, and the cycles of life. Just as the moon moves through its phases, feminine energy is seen as fluid, reflective, and ever-changing. Ancient traditions often linked the moon to goddesses and the nurturing, creative forces of nature. The moon invites us to embrace softness, introspection, and the power of cyclical renewal. Each phase of the moon—from new to full—brings different energetic qualities that we can tap into for growth, healing, and alignment. The period of the new moon is a time for reflection and setting intentions, a moment of inner stillness where new beginnings can take root. As the moon waxes, energy builds, and it's a time for action, growth, and manifestation. The full moon amplifies our emotional state and brings on a culmination of energy, offering a moment of vibrancy. As the moon wanes, it invites introspection, letting go, and clarity. Similarly to the hormonal shifts of the menstrual cycle, the moon's phases can influence our energy and emotional state.

Infradian Rhythms

These are natural biological cycles that occur over a period longer than 24 hours. Both the menstrual cycle and the moon cycle are considered infradian rhythms. These rhythms influence our energy, mood, and productivity, playing a significant role in our overall health and well-being.

Circadian Rhythms

Circadian rhythms occur within an approximately 24-hour cycle and regulate many of our biological processes, including our sleep-wake pattern, hormone release, and body temperature. Often referred to as the body's internal clock, circadian rhythms are influenced by external cues, primarily light and darkness. They help to synchronize various systems in the body with the day-night cycle, optimizing energy levels during specific times of day.

Ultradian Rhythms

Ultradian rhythms are natural cycles that last less than 24 hours and typically range between 90 and 120 minutes. They regulate periods of high and low energy throughout the day, with phases of heightened alertness followed by a dip in energy. These cycles occur multiple times throughout the day, influencing our focus, productivity, and need for rest. For example, after about 90 minutes of intense focus, many people experience a natural dip in energy, signaling the need for a break or a shift in activity. Honoring the ultradian rhythm by taking regular breaks and allowing yourself to rest can improve overall well-being, boost creativity, and help sustain your energy throughout the day.

Seasonal Rhythms

As the seasons change, so do the energies that govern our lives. Understanding the energies of seasonal rhythms can help us deepen our connection with each phase of the menstrual and moon cycles. Winter, with its quiet and introspective energy, invites us to slow down and rest. It's a time for conservation, reflection, and inner work. The darkness and stillness of the season encourages us to recharge, reassess, and restore our energy for the cycle phases ahead. We naturally seek comfort, solitude, and a deeper connection with ourselves, allowing our bodies and minds to rejuvenate before the burst of activity to come. As Winter fades into Spring, a shift in energy occurs. Spring brings renewal, growth, and a fresh beginning. The rising energy encourages creativity, action, and exploration. It's a time to plant seeds for the future. We feel a natural urge to take risks, start new projects, and move forward with fresh enthusiasm. Summer, with its warmth and abundance, amplifies this outward energy. It's a time for expansion, socializing, and embracing the fullness of life. The days are longer and our energy is high, allowing us to express ourselves freely, connect with others, and celebrate the fruits of our efforts. It's a period of productivity and joy, when we seek adventure and experience life to its fullest. As we transition into Fall or Autumn, our energy begins to lessen. This is a time for harvesting and reflection, for letting go of what no longer serves us. The cooler temperatures and shorter days draw us inward, encouraging introspection, completion, and preparation for the quieter months ahead. Fall invites us to tie up loose ends, wrap up projects, and find balance before the pause of Winter returns.

Elemental Energies

The four elemental energies—Water, Air, Fire, and Earth—represent fundamental forces that influence both our inner and outer worlds. While some systems of thought associate water with the Fall (Autumn) season, I align it with Winter, seeing it as a symbol of embryonic waters filled with pure potential—it is a deep metaphysical well from which we can draw. This alignment of water with Winter is in harmony with the Chinese Five Elements system.

Water is the element of emotion, intuition, and flow. It represents the deep currents of our subconscious, guiding us through emotional healing and self-discovery. Water's energy encourages adaptability and emotional intelligence, allowing us to navigate life's challenges with grace and connect with our intuition. Water nurtures creativity and supports healing.

Air, the element of intellect, communication, and inspiration, brings clarity and insight. It encourages us to expand our mind, explore new ideas, and communicate freely. Air's energy fosters creativity and innovation, opening up possibilities and inspiring fresh perspectives.

Fire brings passion, action, and transformation. It fuels our desires and ignites our motivation to pursue our goals with enthusiasm and confidence. Fire's energy pushes us to boldly step into our personal power and create positive change. It represents willpower, vitality, and the courage to leap into new adventures.

Earth offers grounding, stability, and nourishment. It's the energy of practicality and structure, providing a solid foundation. Earth connects us to the physical world and promotes balance, practicality, and a sense of groundedness.

Astrological energies are deeply influenced by the four elements, each of which corresponds to specific signs. Water signs (Cancer, Scorpio, Pisces) are intuitive, emotional, and empathetic, connecting them to their feelings, intuition, and the depths of the subconscious. Air signs (Gemini, Libra, Aquarius) represent intellect, communication, and social connection, and they spark with curiosity, ideas, and a desire for knowledge.

Fire signs (Aries, Leo, Sagittarius) embody passion, action, and creativity, driving them to pursue their desires with enthusiasm and confidence. Earth signs (Taurus, Virgo, Capricorn) are grounded, practical, and reliable, providing stability, structure, and a deep connection to the physical world.

In the tarot card deck, a divination tool, the four suits represent different aspects of life and offer guidance and insight into our personal journey. The Cups suit focuses on emotions, intuition, and relationships. It invites us to explore our inner world, feelings, and the connections we build with others, highlighting themes of love, compassion, and emotional growth. The Swords suit is associated with the mind, intellect, and communication. It highlights our thoughts, decisions, and conflicts, encouraging clarity, truth, and the resolution of mental challenges. The Wands suit represents action, creativity, and passion. It reflects our drive, ambition, and the pursuit of new ideas, encouraging us to take bold steps toward our goals and embrace the energy of inspiration. The Pentacles suit deals with material matters, such as wealth, career, and physical health. It emphasizes the importance of stability, growth, and manifestation, urging us to take practical actions that lead to long-term success and security. Together, the suits in tarot provide a comprehensive framework for understanding the various dimensions of our lives.

What can you glean from exploring the various energies of the cycles, rhythms, and elements? Do you recognize the connections between them? When you consider the influence of the menstrual cycle's follicular phase and compare it with the characteristics of the waxing moon, Spring, the element of Air, the astrological traits of Air signs, and the Swords tarot suit, what do you discover?

The Cycle Magic system integrates cycles, rhythms, and elemental and metaphysical energies to create a dynamic four-phase structure for manifesting. In the following pages, our discussion of each phase is accompanied by practices, exercises, and tools designed to help you align with and amplify the unique energy of that phase. This framework will allow you to manifest the life you desire—one filled with wellness, purpose, and fulfillment.

Chapter 3

HOW CYCLE MAGIC WORKS

• • • • • • • • • •

If you attune yourself to the wisdom within and around you, you'll awaken the clues that will guide you toward your dreams. By choosing to expand and thrive in the process, you'll learn to surrender to the knowing that every step is leading you to where you're meant to be.

The Cycle Magic System

It's time to explore the Cycle Magic system! Beginning with the Attune phase, you'll move through the four phases of energy on your manifesting journey, with each phase having its own unique qualities that you can harness to your advantage. Every phase carries a specific energetic signature, and I'll provide you with practices designed to help you maximize the supportive energy available during that time.

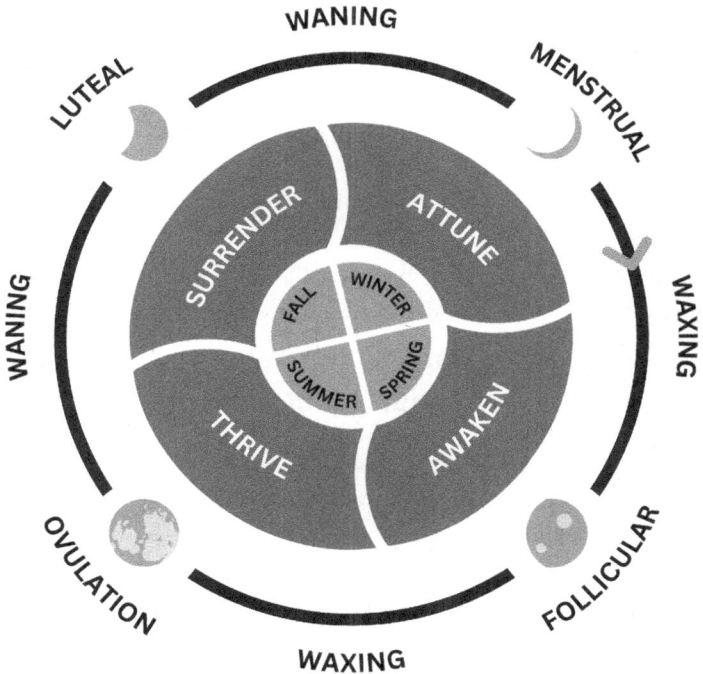

Attune

The Attune phase is the beginning of the cycle, whether aligning with the new moon or the first day of menstruation. This phase holds the energies of Winter, the element of Water, and the energetic attributes of emotion and intuition. It's a time for rest and tapping into your heart and soul desires.

Awaken

This phase aligns with the waxing moon or follicular phase and is imbued with the energies of Spring, the element of Air, and the energetic attributes of intellect and action. It's the perfect time to take action to manifest your heart and soul desires.

Thrive

The culmination of the cycle, the Thrive phase is aligned with the full moon or ovulation. The energies of Summer, the element of Fire, and the energetic attribute of passion drive this phase, helping you confidently embody your manifestations.

Surrender

Offering an opportunity for reflection, this phase aligns with the waning moon or luteal (premenstrual) phase and the energies of Fall, the element of Earth, and the energetic attribute of groundedness. It's a time for inner work, practicality, and detachment.

Should I Align with My Menstrual Cycle or the Moon Cycle?

The first step in your manifesting journey is to decide on which infradian rhythm you prefer to align with—your menstrual cycle or the moon cycle. Take a few grounding deep breaths and read through the tips below to find out which choice feels best for you. There is no right or wrong way to do this. Consider this your first practice in honing your intuition. You can always change your mind for an upcoming cycle, so there's no need to feel locked in.

Menstrual Cycle Tips

- If you are not on hormonal birth control (such as the pill or a patch, implant, injection, ring, hormonal IUD, or another such method of administration) and your cycle is mostly regular, you may want to align with your menstrual cycle as your first choice. If you use hormonal birth control you can choose to align with either your menstrual cycle or the moon cycle, as you prefer. You can always change your mind for future cycles. Choose what feel best for you right now.

- Your full cycle journey will take the same number of days as your menstrual cycle. This on average will be around 28 days, but could be anywhere from 21 to 35 days.

- Use a tracking system to predict your period and ovulation—this will come in handy for aligning with each phase. See "Resources" on page 264 for suggestions.

- Your Cycle Magic journey will begin with the Attune phase around Day 1 of your cycle, the first day of menstruation. You may begin a day or two before or after Day 1 of your cycle if it's more convenient for you. For example, if your period begins on a busy Friday and Saturday is free of commitments, you can engage with the Attune phase practices on Saturday (Day 2 of your period). There is room for flexibility.

Moon Cycle Tips

- Find a website or app that you like to track the phases of the moon. See "Resources" on page 264 for suggestions, or do an online search for moon phase tracking.

- There are four main occurrences to look for when aligning with the moon cycle: the dates of the new moon, first quarter moon, full moon, and last quarter moon. These are milestones you can use to orient yourself as you journey through the four main phases of the moon cycle. Your full cycle journey will take approximately 29 days.

- Align with the phases as closely as you can, but don't worry about being exact. The new moon and full moon phases are short, and can be observed for approximately 2 to 3 days. Between the new moon and full moon, you will have approximately 12 to 14 days to engage with the Awaken phase tools and exercises, and similarly, between the full moon and the new moon you will have 12 to 14 days to engage with the Surrender phase materials.

- Begin your journey with the Attune phase around the time of the new moon. You may begin a day or two before or after the exact date of the new moon if it's more convenient for your schedule. For example, if the new moon is due to appear on a Monday that will be a busy day at work, you might prefer to take time on the Sunday before to engage with the Attune phase practices.

Whether you begin at the new moon or on the first day of your cycle, your first activity in the Attune phase will be the Heart and Soul Desires Meditation on page 63. Because the entire Cycle Magic system supports the journey of bringing your heart and soul desires into manifestation, this is an important first step. We have to know what we want before we can manifest it.

For each of the four phases—Attune, Awaken, Thrive, and Surrender—I've recommended two or three of the provided exercises. You can try them during your very first cycle, and then feel free to revisit them in future cycles if you wish. After the recommended exercises in each phase are additional practices that you can dip into during future cycles. The Cycle Magic system is a lifelong guide for manifesting that you engage with monthly, so there are *plenty* of practices to meet you where you are each time you journey through a particular phase.

I'm sure you're curious about all the Cycle Magic practices, so to get a feel for what's coming up, feel free to read through them before getting started with the Attune phase. Be sure to bookmark your favorites for use during your upcoming cycle. Some practices will be heart-centering and replenishing, some will be fun and creative, and some will ask you to dig a little deeper in self-reflection. Each tiny internal shift you make can have profound effects in your external world. You'll find that there's a time for everything—rest, aligned action, celebration, self-care, and more. You *can* have it all—just not all at once. The support the Cycle Magic system provides will guide you so you can flow with magnetic, intuitive, powerful feminine energy. To get the most out of the Cycle Magic system, be sure to use the exercises, tools, and practices—that will bring them alive and into your world, giving you the best chances of attracting what you desire. Have a journal or notebook ready for use with the inner-work exercises in each phase. The key to manifesting is the *embodiment* of the teachings and practices, so set aside some time during each phase to delve into the practices.

This is *your* journey of manifestation, so I invite you to tweak anything to make it work better for you, whether it's to use a practice in a different phase than I've suggested, or even to create your own practices!

PART II

THE CYCLE MAGIC SYSTEM

Chapter 4

ATTUNE

• • • • • • • • •

> **Moon Phase:** New Moon and Waxing Crescent
> **Menstrual Phase:** Menstruation
> **Season:** Winter
> **Element:** Water
> **Energetic Attributes:** Emotion and Intuition
> **Essence:** Potential, ethereal, spiritual, concealed, embryonic, imagination, space, pause, attract, restore, void, limitless, stillness, rest, regenerate, unseen, inward, fluid

The expansive void of the moonless night sky, the retreating Winter light, the fluidity of emotions, and the deep intuition linked to menstruation all provide clues about the energies available in this phase. The ethereal ripples of the unseen realm beckon you inward toward self-reflection and eventually self-mastery.

Coaching client Ashley was in her thirties and looking to improve her work-life balance when we began working together to support her wellness goals. She had a busy life and was naturally energetic and active. A multitasking maven, she managed a small advertising sales team, arranged weekly networking events, and loved to take her niece and nephew out to sports games on weekends. As a result of her always-on-the-go lifestyle, she was prone to snacking on processed foods and needed support in creating an evening routine to wind down her busy mind and body in preparation for a good night's sleep—something she struggled to get.

But just as Ashley began adopting some of the healthy habits I recommended, something unexpected happened. A collision on a ski slope during a weekend trip resulted in a compression fracture that meant that she had to wear a back brace and rest for a few months while her spine healed. For Ashley, this was devastating news. Although the pain was manageable, she felt trapped and unable to pursue the things she cared about and keep up with her busy lifestyle. As someone who was often revved up on caffeine and adrenaline, she grew frustrated and angry because of her forced immobility. In a coaching session, she told me she replayed the accident over and over in her mind, admonishing herself for not being more careful. Although she was able to take paid time off from her job, she was overcome by worry about losing momentum in her career and endangering her chances of advancement. This mindset had a domino effect and began to derail her efforts to make healthier choices. Ashley was fighting the situation she was in with so much resistance that it was causing heightened levels of anxiety—quite the opposite of her doctor's orders to rest and heal.

I offered her a concept to consider that might help her mindset. "Ashley, what if this is your long-overdue personal season of Winter?"

She paused and quietly asked me what I meant by "personal season of Winter."

"It sounds like you've been living this fast-paced, on-the-go lifestyle that doesn't seem sustainable long-term. What if you viewed the doctor's order to rest as a prescription from the

Universe to take a break from your usual pace in life and try a different way of living, temporarily, in order to heal and restore?" She agreed that her hectic lifestyle did get overwhelming at times, and that she had been saving up for a vacation.

"Ashley, what if this is a time to not only heal your spine, but also heal the anxiety and stress that have been interfering with your sleep and eating habits? What if you *fully embrace* your personal season of Winter, with the anticipation that Spring is just around the corner?"

Ashley was on board. "Okay. . . . How do I do that, exactly?"

The secret is, it's more about *being* than doing. I suggested that Ashley embrace the aspects of Winter that felt deeply soothing to her mind, body, and soul. "Ooh, like fuzzy socks, vegetable soups, meditation, and reading?" she asked.

Ashley was right on track, and in addition to these cozy Winter comforts, she also spent time detaching from technology, creating a mood board of her goals, reflecting and journaling on her thoughts and emotions, experimenting with essential oils, soaking up the sun in her garden, giving herself gua sha facials, and making friendship bracelets with her niece. She reduced her intake of caffeine, did some gentle physical therapy, and adopted an approach of self-compassion for her mind and body. Ashley no longer berated herself about the accident. Instead, she treated herself with patience and kindness. Like the steam that rose from her evening mug of herbal tea, any resistance to her situation evaporated. And in the midst of relishing her season of Winter, Ashley received a report from her doctor that her healing was on track. It would soon be time to emerge from the self-care cocoon and enter the world again, but in a new and better way.

This was a time of soul-searching and self-discovery for Ashley. She realized that her dreams were not something to chase externally, but to connect with internally. She no longer felt pressure to try to fit everything into her busy days. She was ready with her heart-centered plan of action to take her dreams forward. This time, she would create a monthly ritual to rest for a couple of days and attune her mind and body with her soul for the deep replenishment she craved.

Reflecting on her long-overdue personal season of Winter, Ashley shared with me, "You know what's funny? The vacation I was working so hard to save up for was at a remote retreat where they serve healthy meals, offer meditation sessions and spa treatments, and give you time to spend in nature. I feel like I just saved thousands of dollars and had a similar experience right here at home!"

There is a season for everything, and the Attune phase is your season to embrace the opportunity for rest and rejuvenation, while the supportive energetic influences help you connect with deep wisdom and soul revelations. Both menstruation and the new moon have long been associated with the energies of stillness, rest, and heightened intuition. Once revered, this magical feminine power later became shrouded and shamed, and the world started beating to the drum of the daily masculine energy cycle. By rediscovering the metaphysical gifts that can be tapped into during the Attune phase, we can appreciate this regular connection with rest and learn to move within more of a monthly rhythm that will become instinctual and act as a supportive structure for manifesting the lives we truly want to live.

In nature, the new moon aligns with periods of rest or reclusiveness for several types of animals. Some migratory birds and nocturnal mammals are less active during the new moon's darkness, choosing this phase as a time to retreat. The ancient agricultural practice of lunar gardening recognizes the new moon as the beginning of a new growth cycle. Seeds planted at this time are believed to benefit from the moon's gravitational pull, which draws water to the surface, increasing soil moisture. Rising moisture, along with the gentle influence of the moon's growing light, encourages the next phase of growth.

The Attune phase is also associated with Winter, the darkest season. The darkness, the void, the stillness, the undefined, can be daunting or even scary. There is a limitless quality to nothingness. Like the soil, the substrate, the embryonic liquid life emerges from. It is undefinable, until such time that our consciousness chooses to define it. It's a kind of blank canvas on which to sketch your dreams. A movie screen to project your desires onto.

This is a time when we can access our subconscious mind and imprint it with our desired manifestations. The subconscious plays a profound role in shaping our thoughts, behaviors, and overall well-being. It operates below the surface of our conscious awareness, influencing how we perceive and interpret the world around us. During the Attune phase, we can tap in to the power of the subconscious to reprogram outdated thought patterns and cultivate a more positive mindset that can help us manifest our desires.

The subconscious mind is also closely linked to our emotions and beliefs. By transforming our underlying beliefs and emotional blocks (I call it "alchemizing"—more on that later), we can harness the power of our subconscious and unlock our full potential to create the life we desire.

The season of Winter is also strongly associated with dampness and the element of water. As we find in astrology, tarot, and other spiritual traditions, water is symbolic of emotions. The darkness of the night sky, the expansiveness and liquidity of water, and the intangible realm of emotions—these all hold a limitless, fluid energy. This is the energetic signature of the Attune phase, one of limitless potential.

Intentionally pausing your externally focused, frenetic life, whether for an hour or two or a couple of days, invites in the opportunity to reconnect with the true essence of your existence. It's here, in the Attune phase, where you can embrace rest and stillness to uncover and align with your heart and soul desires.

This chapter offers a potent series of inner-work exercises that will illuminate your deepest truths and support you in setting clear intentions for what you desire to manifest. Within the shadow of the Attune phase, you will recognize and explore any internal resistance to your desires, alchemize limiting thoughts, and imprint your subconscious with new, positive expectations. Once your desires and intentions are cleansed and crystallized, you can broadcast them out into the cosmos through emanation and visualization. On your journey to transform your deepest desires into reality, Attune is your galactic START HERE signpost, and the first step in the manifestation cycle.

Now that we've explored the energetic signature of the Attune phase, how do you feel about it? If it seems too quiet, heavy, or boring, examine this idea. Perhaps it's inviting you into a much-needed space of deep rest and rebalancing, and that may scare you. Just as we wouldn't head to the nearest beach in our bikini in the middle of Winter and complain about the lack of warmth and sunshine, we cannot expect to function at peak performance in the long term without resting, recharging, and reconnecting with our intuitive superpowers. Did you know that adequate sleep and downtime help to regulate our hormones, lower cortisol levels, improve insulin sensitivity, and support balanced energy? This makes it easier to lose excess weight, reduce stress, and maintain our overall wellness.

By embracing the quietude of the Attune phase each month, just as we embrace the season of Winter each year, we can check in with ourselves and continuously reroute our manifesting journey toward soul-aligned goals that fulfill our purpose. Setting strong internal intentions can create seismic external shifts. We slow down in order to fast-track our results. Sure, Winter can be a little heavy and challenging at times, but it also offers us the opportunity to retreat and create a cozy space in which to relax and restore. As I write this, I happen to be embracing the Attune cocoon after gathering all my dearest writing essentials—blue-light-blocking glasses, my favorite lip balm, a chai latte, and fluffy slippers. I have soft background music playing and essential oils being diffused as I sit on my PEMF chair mat for grounding and gaze out at the evening landscape under a sliver of waxing crescent moon. So light a candle, grab a warming beverage and your journal, and let's fully embrace this internally focused phase (adorned with fairy lights, if you wish) so that we may plant the metaphysical seeds of our manifestations in time for them to awaken and flourish in the Spring and beyond.

Where to Begin

It's time to pull up your calendar and decide on the date when you will begin! If you have a natural menstrual cycle and are not currently using a hormonal contraceptive, the best time to begin will be Day 1 of your cycle—your first day of menstruation. Alternatively, it is just as effective to start your manifesting journey on the day of the next new moon. There are several apps and websites that track the moon phases, so doing a little research to find out the date of the next new moon will allow you to plan to begin on that day (see "Resources" on page 264 for suggested apps and websites).

In the pages to come there are three exercises that flow in sequence to help you make the most of this phase, followed by a section called "Attune Phase Practices" that includes additional, optional practices and tools you may also want to explore in future cycles. They are not intended to be used all at once, but rather revisited in future cycles, to keep things interesting, although if you have plenty of time for your first Attune phase exploration, then feel free to dive into as many of the additional practices as you'd like to. It's your toolbox of options, so choose the ones that feel good in the moment. For your very first journey into the Attune phase, however, start with these three core exercises:

1. Heart and Soul Desires Meditation
2. Journaling: Your Heart and Soul Inquiry
3. Create Your Personal Mantras

If you can't complete this sequence of three exercises, that's perfectly okay. If you have to choose just one to do in this phase, make it the Heart and Soul Desires Meditation to uncover your deepest desires, and then jot down what you uncovered in your journal. Allow 15 to 20 minutes for the meditation. I've provided a guided meditation audio file at CycleMagic.com/meditation that's 12:34 minutes long (that was truly a coincidence!) that I recommend listening to if you can, but a meditation transcript is also available here if you prefer to read through the meditation steps, memorize the basic journey of tapping in to your heart and soul desires and complete it in your own time.

It's Time to Attune!

Welcome to Day 1 of your manifesting cycle. Your journey begins here. Ideally, you will be starting on the first day of menstruation if you are aligning with your natural menstrual cycle or on the first day of the new moon if you are aligning with the moon cycle. Let's dive in to the first of the three core exercises of the Attune phase.

What If I Can't Begin on Day 1?

The strongest energies of the Attune phase span approximately three days, with subtler energies being felt on either side of that period as the transition between phases takes place. This is similar to the transitions of day to night and back to day again. Think of Attune as a night that spans seventy-two hours (three days), with a sunset transition period right before full darkness and a sunrise transition period right after full darkness. So if you choose to start your personal Day 1 earlier or later than the "actual" Day 1 of the menstrual or moon cycle, that's okay too! Life happens, and sometimes it makes more sense to spend a restful Sunday diving in to your Attune phase practices than a busy Monday. Allow your intuition to be your guide. So often we look outside of ourselves for the security of a concrete answer, or we have an urge to do things perfectly. Attune is *your* portal for developing your internal superpowers of intuition, self-awareness, confidence, direction, and inner wisdom, and these qualities are so much more powerful than the pursuit of perfection, so deciding to feel good about whatever day you choose to begin your manifesting journey on will serve you well.

1. Heart and Soul Desires Meditation

What are heart and soul desires? You can think of them as cherished dreams, wants, and needs that live deep inside us. They're subtle whispers that softly draw your attention. As we navigate today's fast-paced world, it's easy to overlook or undervalue them. These desires might feel like things we don't quite deserve, or like they belong to some distant future. Sometimes they get crowded out by the more immediate needs and pressures of everyday life. If we feel a twinge of envy when we see someone else living their dream life, it could be a sign that our own long-held desires have been sidelined in favor of actions more aligned with survival. Perhaps we've been so caught up in just getting by that we've forgotten what truly lights us up. We might even feel like although everything's okay, something is missing from our lives—there's an undercurrent of longing that just won't go away. We could assume that our truest desires just won't happen for us, or that their fulfillment is left up to fate. The truth is that our heart and soul desires have the power to break through those walls of doubt and resistance. They can start drawing our dreams to us faster than we might imagine. Our souls are connected to an infinite wellspring of unrealized potential that's waiting for us to tap into it.

If you're ready to get in touch with your true desires, it starts with removing the noise, tapping in, and listening with curiosity to your heart and soul so you can clarify their messages. It took me 15 years of sporadic attempts and practice to allow myself to trust the visions, thoughts, words, and images that I came to experience in meditation. The secret is that what you experience in a guided meditation can be closely linked to your imagination. If you can *imagine* a loving message from your heart and sense whether it feels true, you are doing it right.

Heart energy is very powerful. Science is only just beginning to understand the effects of the electromagnetic field produced by the heart, but it is now clear that the heart actually sends more signals to the brain than the brain sends to the heart. According to the HeartMath Institute, there is evidence that the information contained in the heart's powerful field may play a vital synchronizing role in the body—and affect others around us as well.[1] Rigorous electrophysiological studies have indicated that the heart also appears to play a key role in intuition. What better time is there to tap into our hearts than during the Attune phase?

Preparing for the Heart and Soul Desires Meditation

You are about to embark on a beautiful guided journey to connect with your heart and soul desires and to have the opportunity to be imbued with Divine love and gather the threads of your innermost wishes. Here are some tips to help you prepare:

- **Mind.** Choose a quiet 20-minute window when you are least likely to be interrupted. Switch off any devices that may beep and release any distracting thoughts onto paper to revisit later. Have a pen and your journal ready.

- **Body.** Create a relaxing, dreamy space. Set the mood with soft lighting. You may want to grab a soft throw or cushion and wear comfortable clothing. Do a light stretch or exercise to release any tension in your body before beginning. Try squeezing your muscles and then releasing them. Roll your shoulders forward and backward and shake out your arms and legs.

- **Soul.** Create a sacred portal by energetically clearing the space. Remove any clutter. You may wish to burn sage, incense, or palo santo or to use a sound bowl to clear the energy. You can place your favorite crystal, spiritual book, special item, or oracle card nearby. Consider playing soft spiritual music or binaural beats while you set up the space.

Meditation: A Guided Journey to Your Heart and Soul Desires

This meditation is available as a downloadable audio file at cyclemagic.com/meditation.

1. Begin by getting comfortable and relaxed. Try sitting in a chair with your journal or lie down with your eyes closed if you're using the audio version. Make sure your arms and legs aren't crossed.

2. Feel yourself relax. Release any tension in your jaw, neck, and shoulders.

3. Take a deep, full breath in. Hold it for three seconds and slowly release it. Do this three times. Repeat this affirmation in your mind:

   I am relaxed. I am safe. I am supported. I ask for Divine protection as I take this journey inward.

4. Drop your awareness into your heart space. Begin to sense the pulse of Divine universal love emanating from your heart. Your heart chakra is a portal for Divine love to flow through you. Feel it now as a soft, warm glow of pure love. When you feel into this soft, loving vibration, allow yourself to lightly smile and connect with its bliss.

5. Using the power of your imagination, gently enlarge this glow of love from your heart space and watch as it fills your body. Imagine that every cell of your body is glowing with this universal Divine love energy. Does it feel warm, peaceful, or vibrant? What color is this energy? Bask in its love. Allow it to imbue every part of you. Invite it to dwell in your every dimension. Ask it

to flood your being and soak into the parts that need it the most right now.

6. Love is your birthright and your essence. It's an infinite energy, and as it fills you up, you can also offer this channel of Divine love to others. Love is not a limited energy source that you need to ration from your own energy field, it's an ever-abundant stream of energy that channels through you. See your heart chakra now as an infinite well and channel of Divine love. You no longer need to seek a source of love from outside yourself, it's stirring within you, and you are always able to tune in and connect with it.

7. Ask your heart: *Beautiful heart, my portal to Divine love, what messages do you have for me?* Take a moment to receive any messages; feel free to write them down, or stay in a meditative state.

8. Let's go a little deeper. *Beautiful heart, what are you craving right now? What are your desires?* Pause and listen, noting in your journal or your mind anything that comes up. Thank your heart for the messages you received.

9. From this sacred space of love, journey a little further beyond the body and into your soul realm. Begin to sense your soul as a driving force—your highest self, the part of yourself from which your grandest desires emanate. Know that you have a unique and special soul. Your soul is eternal. It's wise, compassionate, and the expansive part of you that whispers to you. Right now, you are holding space for your soul to communicate with you with clarity, purity, and purpose.

10. It's time for your soul inquiry. Ask: *Beautiful, expansive soul, what are you craving?* Pause to receive any messages and either write them down or remain in your meditative state.

11. Let's go a little deeper. *Beautiful soul, what have you been trying to teach me? What do you need me to see and hear? I receive your message now.* Pause and listen. Thank your soul for its profound messages and invite it to reveal itself more often in your life.

12. Take a moment to recall the messages you received from your heart and your soul. What desires emerged? Visualize them now. What do you desire from your heart and your soul? Do you desire a more loving relationship? The freedom to create? Greater abundance? To be vibrant and well? To experience more harmony? To feel cared for and supported? Or just to be at ease in the flow of life? Whatever it is, imagine that your desires are manifesting before your eyes.

13. Take some time to soak up these good feelings and experience them in your body. How would you *feel* if these desires were manifested? Take a deep breath in and release it. Feel the relief in your body as you accept these gifts into your life. Feel lighter, freer, happier, and all the other feelings that the manifestation of your desires bring you. Imagine that it has all unfolded. Welcome it into the present moment. How very grateful you feel. Your body is so relaxed and at the same time brimming with joy and vibrancy. Allow a smile to come to your face and feel a deep gratitude.

14. It's now time to come back to the here and now. Take a deep breath, and exhale. Become aware of the noises

around you—in the room or outside the room. Breathe deeply, and then gently wiggle your fingers and toes. When you are ready, open your eyes and take as much time as you need to get into a seated position.

2. Journaling: Your Heart and Soul Inquiry

Following the Heart and Soul Desires Meditation, grab your journal and spend some time contemplating these questions. Write as much as you wish; let it flow out of you and onto the paper.

1. What desires do you feel from your heart?
2. What desires do you feel from your soul?

If you didn't receive any messages while you were meditating, that's perfectly fine! Meditation is a practice like anything else, and as you practice, you will learn to open up to the voice inside you. Journaling can also be a great way to wake up that voice, which may have lain dormant for a long time. Begin writing out what you think your desires might be and see where it takes you.

3. Create Your Personal Mantras

My very first experience with using positive affirmations and mantras was during the time I was applying for a U.S. Green Card (a permanent resident card). I had dreamed of living in America ever since I was a small child growing up in Sydney, Australia. Living in London at the time, I applied for the Green Card lottery as one of my first experiments in manifesting. Eight months after applying I received a letter in the mail stating that "all winners have already been contacted by mail," and if I hadn't received the confirmation letter, then my application wasn't successful. Although I felt a little deflated by this news, life was getting pretty good in London. I had begun studying spirituality and meditation, left a relationship that wasn't healthy, changed jobs, and built new friendships with like-minded, spiritual people. It was an exciting time, and I was preparing to move to a modern high-rise apartment overlooking the Thames river.

A few months after moving I received a large envelope that had been forwarded from my previous address. As I opened it, I could hardly believe what I saw. It was a package from the U.S. Embassy in London congratulating me on my successful application for a U.S. Green Card! Somehow, someway, I had won the U.S. Green Card lottery after all. But it wasn't official yet—there was a long list of documents that needed to be submitted to the embassy by September 29. That was only two months away! Although the letter was dated in March, I hadn't received it until July.

The next two months turned out to be a marathon of manifesting practices as I applied all the positive-thinking and manifesting tools I was learning toward making this dream come true. This entailed waking up in the middle of the night to call a government office in Australia to try to convince a young man named Luke to send me a copy of my police background report even though I'd mistakenly sent them a check for ten dollars more than the required amount. On the call, Luke insisted that their policy would not allow him to process the check and that he would need to receive a new check before they could run the report and send me a copy. I sighed and told him I would mail him a new check, knowing full well that there just wasn't enough time for this document to be processed and mailed to me in time to submit it to the embassy in London before the September 29 deadline.

After the call, I stayed up until all hours of the night and meditated. I repeated positive affirmations. I connected with spiritual books and tools, and I visualized that my U.S. Green Card was coming to fruition. The next day I spoke to my dad in Sydney, and he agreed to mail Luke at the government office a check in the correct amount to cover the report I needed. This would cut the time down by a lot, and at this point, every day mattered. After several more post-midnight calls to Luke, followed by late-night meditation and affirmation sessions, he reluctantly agreed to receive a check from my dad on my behalf, even though this was against their policy. The background report from Australia was finally in process. But would it be mailed to me in time to get it to the U.S. Embassy in London by the September 29 deadline?

I continued my nightly sessions of meditation, affirmations, and envisioning a positive outcome. I visualized myself visiting family in New York, and breathing in fresh ocean air in California. On Monday, September 25, I still hadn't received the report in the mail from Australia, but I took positive action in spite of this. The only way to submit documents to the U.S. Embassy was by a private courier that had to be booked one day in advance. Although the background report hadn't physically arrived yet, I went ahead and booked the courier for a pickup on Wednesday the 27th. When the report still hadn't shown up by that date, I rebooked the courier for Thursday, the 28th of September. When the report still didn't show up in the mail by the morning of Thursday the 28th, I confidently rebooked it for the following day, Friday, September 29—my final chance.

I had held on so tightly to this dream of living in America, and now I had to face the possibility that it might not work out. It was sad to think that I'd come *this close* to manifesting my desire, especially after putting so much energy and intention into it. I spoke to a friend that day, and he reminded me that "energy is never wasted," a spiritual concept I'd been learning about. Energy doesn't just disappear, it transforms. I believe that all the positivity, effort, good wishes, belief, and actions that we channel toward a dream simply have to show up *somewhere* in our lives. This mirrors the law of conservation of energy in physics, which states that energy in a closed system can neither be created nor destroyed.[2] Perhaps it transforms into something that shows up in a different or better way than we expected? I pondered this thought as I went home that evening and checked my mailbox one last time, finally willing to relinquish my long-held desire if the Universe simply had a better plan for me. And there it was.

Part of manifesting your heart and soul desires entails energetically "stepping into" the identity of the future version of you—the version who *naturally* has these manifestations happen in her life. Visualize her now, and step into that identity. It's time to create a few mantras based on your heart and soul desires that connect with this next-level, empowered version of you! Personal mantras, or positive affirmations, work by influencing the subconscious mind, leading to positive impacts on both the brain and body. When we craft personal mantras, we are helping to orient our energy toward our desires in a powerful way. Imagine someone with a blindfold on standing in the middle of a darkened room. Now imagine that you know where the door is, but the only thing you are allowed to do to help them is to gently rotate their body so they are facing in the direction of the door. Your input, although seemingly subtle, would be a huge help to them in being able to find a way out to the light. Mantras and affirmations work in a similar way to direct our subconscious mind.

Repeating our mantras encourages new neural pathways to form in the brain, making it easier to maintain positive thinking—and leading to positive actions. This change is known as *neuroplasticity*. Research shows that affirmations can also reduce stress and boost self-confidence and overall sense of well-being.[3] The more often we repeat our personal mantras, the more we strengthen our mindset, break self-sabotaging habits, and move in the direction of achieving our goals.

Mantras are most powerful when they are written in the present tense, as opposed to being framed as something you hope happens in the future. Remember, you are stepping into the future version of yourself *now*. By writing your personal mantras in present tense, you bring the future into the present. You'll want to create mantras that are:

Personal: They hold great meaning for you and your life.

Powerful: They excite and motivate you.

Positive: They feel uplifting.

Present: They are written in the present tense.

Write down 5 to 10 powerful "I am" statements that define the new you. Here are some examples to get you started:

I am healthy and full of vitality.

I am a magnet for abundance.

I am feeling more confident every day.

I am happy and share my joy with others.

I am loved and able to give and receive love freely.

Now, it is time to create your personal mantras. Craft mantras that feel good to you, and then write them in your journal or here.

1.

2.

3.

4.

5.

6.

7.

8.

9.

10.

Now that you've come up with some powerful mantras, let's explore the best ways to employ these little helpers so they can imprint your subconscious mind and help to orient you in the direction of your dreams. Here are three ways to access your subconscious mind:

1. **Repetition.** Repeat affirmative statements and mantras over and over so your subconscious mind learns to record those thoughts, as it does for any important regularly recurring thought or experience.[4] Set an alarm that alerts you to do this at intervals throughout the day. This could be every two hours during waking hours, or at 3 P.M., 6 P.M., and 9 P.M. When your alarm

goes off, spend a few minutes repeating your mantras over and over.

2. **Sleep.** Just before falling asleep or immediately upon waking, the mind is shifting gears and the subconscious mind is more accessible,[5] so repeat your mantras as you fall asleep and as you wake up. This sounds easy, but it can take some practice, so keep persisting. You could also record your mantras and play them back as you fall asleep.

3. **Daydreaming.** The subconscious mind is also more accessible when we are daydreaming, or when our mind starts to wander as we do simple, repetitive tasks like cleaning dishes, watering plants, or brushing our teeth. When you catch yourself going into autopilot and your mind starts to wander, begin repeating your mantras. Placing notes at locations near where you perform daily routines can help to remind you.

Your challenge is to repeat your empowering personal mantras over and over again as much as you can, especially when your subconscious mind is more accessible. It takes practice, but the rewards are worth the effort. This is a powerful tool that can help you to manifest your dreams!

Rewiring the Subconscious Brain

You may be asking, "What makes it possible to alter our subconscious mind while we fall asleep or engage in repetitive tasks?" The answer is theta waves. Lecturer and biologist Dr. Bruce Lipton teaches that our subconscious mind is particularly receptive to new information twice a day—upon waking and when falling asleep. This happens when our brains operate at a "theta" vibrational frequency. Over a 24-hour period, our brains go through different states, like deep sleep (delta frequency); falling asleep, dreaming, or waking up from a deep sleep (theta frequency); awake but relaxed (alpha frequency); alert and engaged (beta frequency); and intensely thinking (gamma frequency). The theta frequency, associated with intuition, creativity, and healing, occurs as we wake from deep sleep, and as we fall asleep. Even though our conscious mind shuts down during this transition, the subconscious remains active. This is the perfect time for reprogramming the subconscious mind by repeating our mantras. As a bonus, repeating mantras and affirmations while drifting off to sleep has been shown to aid in falling asleep quicker. This is thought to happen because we reduce our "mind chatter" when we focus on a mantra or affirmation. When we engage in repetitive tasks and find ourselves operating on autopilot and daydreaming, once again we are in theta wave territory. Being in this frequency has other benefits as well. We can not only imprint our subconscious mind with positive mantras, but also generate creative ideas and shortcuts to help us manifest things. Have you ever had a brilliant idea or a solution to a problem come to you while you were in the shower? Or how about while driving? Or walking in a park? If so, you're not alone. Many great thought leaders and organizations over the centuries have realized the benefits of tapping into this realm. According to some reports, while working on the theory of relativity, Albert Einstein would lie down to rest to allow inspiration for his work to arise. While living in London in my 20s, I had the opportunity to work for an innovations agency. Our team worked with clients like Microsoft, Unilever, Hasbro, Virgin, and Ben & Jerry's to help them build cultures of creativity and innovation. We facilitated brainstorming sessions to guide their brand managers in coming up with hundreds of new product ideas, and each year we hosted a big conference for our global clients. The theme of the conference one particular year was "The Garden Shed," based on the premise that when we spend time puttering around on nonurgent tasks (like gardening or tinkering with tools or crafts), we switch over to the theta brain frequency, and *that* is when innovative ideas can propagate. With some of the world's most productive and innovative companies recognizing the value of leveraging the human brain's potential for creative magic, it also seems worth exploring within the realm of manifesting.

Attune Phase Practices

What follows is a collection of optional activities for you to incorporate into your Attune phases going forward. As you become more and more familiar with the energy of this phase, you might want to add your own ideas and exercises to this selection. Think of this as a menu where you can pick and choose which practices resonate with you and delve into them around your time of menstruation if you're following your menstrual cycle or around the time of the new moon if you're following the moon cycle. This is when the natural universal energies best support our inner-work practices. You might also like to try some of these out during the season of Winter, or really at any time when the mood strikes. Or keep things simple and try just one of these practices each time you arrive at your Attune phase (about once a month).

Clarifying Your Heart and Soul Desires

Depending on what your experience was with the Heart and Soul Desires Meditation, you may have abstract, vague, broad, or half-formed ideas about what your desires actually are. If this is the case, you may need to give them further attention and expansion to make them clearer and more real. When we take a broad desire and begin asking the question *how?* it helps us drill down and get more clarity. You can use the word *how* as a tool to explore your desires more deeply.

In this exercise you will revisit your heart and soul desires and explore ways of writing them out in more specific detail by asking how you can make them clearer. You could also think of this as setting intentions for how you will go about manifesting a particular desire. Here is an example:

> **Heart and Soul Desire:** To feel more alive
>
> **HOW could you feel more alive in your life?** By feeling healthier and more vibrant
>
> **HOW could you feel healthier and more vibrant?** By eating healthy and working out
>
> **HOW do you intend to eat healthy and work out?** By eating organic, eating one raw meal a day, trying yoga or Pilates, doing a fun cardio workout three times a week, eating more superfoods, detoxing twice a year, joining my friend at their workout class, buying some light weights for home workouts, going hiking on a local trail on Sundays, quitting refined sugar, trying two weeks gluten-free, following fitness instructors on social media for inspiration

Do you see that by using the word *how* you can get more specific about your desire each time you ask another *how* question? Here is another example.

Heart and Soul Desire: To feel more secure

HOW can you feel more secure? By knowing I won't lose my home

HOW could you know that you won't lose your home? By having enough money

HOW do you intend to have enough money? By keeping a security fund of six months' living expenses, by going for a promotion and salary increase at work, by updating my résumé and applying for better-paying jobs, by learning a new skill and starting a side business, by asking friends if they know of any opportunities that can help me earn more, by monetizing the creative hobbies I enjoy on weekends, by learning more about how to invest, by maximizing my 401(k), by sticking to my budget each month

In most cases, by the first or second time you ask *how*, you will have a clear picture of what your desire is and you can stop there. I've taken these examples to the next stage of detail just to illustrate the power of this exercise, but you don't need to take it that far. You can simply ask one *how* message at a time until your desire becomes clearer to you. If you want to try this, grab your journal and explore how you can bring your desire into greater focus.

If you feel that your desires are already quite specific, you can skip this exercise and choose a different one. However, if you are curious and want to explore why a very specific desire came up, try asking why. This will help you zoom out and understand the underlying essence of your heart and soul desires. Here is an example.

Heart and Soul Desire: To get a dog

WHY do you want to do that? To care for it, and to know it will be there for me

WHY is that important? So I can give and receive love

WHY do you want to do that? To feel more love in my life

Here is another example.

Heart and Soul Desire: To travel to Costa Rica

WHY do you want to do that? To allow myself to connect with nature

WHY is that important? To relax and enter a meditative state

WHY do you like that? To fill myself with appreciation

WHY is that important? To feel a close connection with a higher power

Notice that by using the word *why*, you can get a bigger-picture view of your specific desire each time you ask another *why* question. This is also a great exercise to do if your desire was to have more money. When we reflect on *why* we want more money, it can bring us clarity about the things in life that we truly desire.

By playing the *how* and *why* game with your desires and zooming in and out like a microscope, you can really get a sense of what is important to you, why it is important, and how you can better understand the desire. This level of self-knowledge and clarity can act like a magnet to align you with the things you truly desire and help you to recognize them when they come into your world.

Identifying Your Shadow Messages (Shadow Message Workshop, Part I)

Our cherished heart and soul desires can mean so much to us, but at the same time, for various reasons we may not truly *believe* that they could come into manifestation. Sometimes when we think about the exciting, expansive new manifestations coming into our lives it can be closely followed by thoughts that feel heavier, fearful, or limiting. In this exercise, we will identify those little voices and thoughts that give us resistance. I call these Shadow Messages.

Shadow Messages can be scary, but after we bring them out into the light, we can work to transform them. To do this, after completing this exercise, you may want to take this work a step further—either during the current or a future Attune phase, depending on your schedule. Attune is a rather short phase (about three days), so I've broken this Shadow Message work into two parts to help you make time for it. You can think of this as a workshop split into two sessions to be taken in sequence, but not necessarily at the same time.

In this exercise, we will just focus on *identifying* our Shadow Messages. You may be wondering where these Shadow Messages come from and what their purpose is. In short, they are there to protect us from things like disappointment, failure, exposure, embarrassment, and abandonment. They tend to lurk in the shadows of our subconscious mind. Our subconscious can operate like a recorder of our thoughts and experiences. It collects and archives information that we later draw upon. This is especially true in childhood, when our minds are often in the theta frequency (i.e., connected to the subconscious mind). Before we reach our teenage years, our mind is like a sponge, collecting information without necessarily having the ability to determine if the beliefs we are forming are helpful to our growth or not.

As you can imagine, certain thoughts and beliefs that were imprinted on the subconscious mind years ago are no longer relevant. When it comes to expanding our lives and manifesting new things, chances are we need to rewrite the old records and ditch any outdated fears and limitations to better move forward.

So how do we identify these Shadow Messages? Although they are different for each person, they all tend to have a critical tone and can also feel resistant to change. They can show up as a "reality check" and seem very logical. Here are some examples of what Shadow Messages might sound like:

- Where will I find the time to do this?
- I can't do this without first doing...
- I can't do this alone.
- What if it fails?
- Where do I even begin?
- How will I find the resources I need?
- What will they think if I do this?
- It is not the right time; I should wait until...
- This would be fun, but first I need to prioritize...
- I can't start this right now, I'm too busy.

Do any of these sound familiar? The best way to see what kind of Shadow Messages are holding you back from expanding your comfort zone is to explore them in relation to the desires you wish to manifest—we'll get to that shortly. The messages often promise some kind of comfort or benefit when we listen to them (which is why they are so seductive), but ultimately they keep us stuck.

Like many women, I've attempted to start new fitness regimens over the years, and failed at one after another. On reflection, I can see that certain Shadow Messages that popped up along the way revealed very valid concerns. Some of my Shadow Messages told me that:

- Launching such a high-energy program feels too intense.
- Yoga is boring, so I'm going to lose interest.
- The gyms I like are too expensive.
- I'll need to buy new equipment and workout gear if I choose this workout.
- My workout clothes are not stylish enough.
- Group fitness classes give me anxiety. Once the door closes, you're in it until the end.
- I'm not as fit as everyone else in the class.
- Hiking is dangerous. What if I cross paths with a rattlesnake or a mountain lion?
- I hate carrying a water bottle when I'm walking because they are so heavy.

In the interest of keeping this brief, I'm going to stop here, but trust me, this is the tip of the iceberg when it comes to my fitness-related Shadow Messages. Unfortunately, many of these limiting thoughts stopped me in my tracks and foiled my fitness goals—for years. I didn't take the time to investigate them, hear them out, and rework the proposed workout to suit me better. I didn't invest too much time in self-reflection because external circumstances were busy campaigning for my attention. Here's the thing—external circumstances will always be there. Recently, however, by engaging in a few hours of self-reflection and inner work at least once a month, I've made small but consistent tweaks that have revolutionized my life. My fitness routine today aligns with the natural energy ebb and flow of my menstrual cycle. Depending on what phase I'm in and how I feel on a particular day, I'm engaged in movement in one of a variety of ways—a gentle 20-minute mat Pilates class, a 40-minute session on an indoor bike (while watching a TV show), a walk on a treadmill or along the beach, an online cardio dance class, short sets of lifting weights at home, or a hike in the nearby hills—and so far I haven't run into any mountain lions.

My fitness choices did require some investment in new workout gear, some equipment, and online classes, but I allocated the resources for these in my monthly budget by making a few tweaks and planning my purchases over time. I prioritized my wellness and started building habits of movement into each phase of my cycle (more on that in the next chapter).

I often find that once a person makes a decision to improve an area of their life, resources can be found to help support those new goals. Some of my wellness clients have found creative ways to meet their fitness goals without breaking the bank. This includes working out with a friend who has a gym at their apartment complex, wearing ankle and wrist weights around the house when tidying up, dancing and playing with children, and finding deep discounts for online classes through their health insurance. Are you hearing any Shadow Messages right now? If so, write them down.

When you do that, there's no need to analyze them, or to try to dismiss or justify them. Just notice them and record what's coming up in your journal. The ultimate goal (which is accomplished in Shadow Message Workshop, Part II) is to move through the resistance of these messages and transform them into something helpful. But for now, just work on gathering all your Shadow Messages. They are lurking there, looking kind of scary, but it's time to shine a light on these shadows. Begin by noting down one of the desires you'd like to manifest. This could be one of your heart and soul desires from the meditation earlier in this chapter. Then come up with one action step you could take to help you manifest this desire. Listen for and write down the Shadow Messages that follow.

Steps:

Desire: What is it that you desire to manifest?
Action: What action could you take to help make it happen?
Shadow Messages: What Shadow Messages come up?

Example 1:

Desire: To feel healthier
Action: Spend one day a week going to a fitness class with my friend
Shadow Messages: What if I can't keep up with the rest of the class? What if everyone there is super fit and I look like the odd one out? What if I bump into someone from work when I'm all sweaty?

Example 2:

Desire: To follow my passion

Action: Start a social media channel on a topic I'm passionate about
Shadow Messages: What if I don't get many followers? The proper equipment is probably too expensive. What if my parents/my ex/someone from work sees it? What if people leave negative comments?

Example 3:

Desire: To find love
Action: Go on a dating site and be open to going on dates
Shadow Messages: At my age, there are no great partners left. Dating sites are so cringe; it feels like I'm desperate. What if I get catfished by someone with a fake profile? What if I like someone and they end up ghosting me? What if I land a date but then they stand me up?

Grab your journal, take a deep breath, and go ahead and confront your Shadow Messages. This is brave inner work you are doing, and though it may feel overwhelming, remember—you are just putting these thoughts down on paper. Getting them out of your head frees you up to see them clearly and release them. You're doing great!

Alchemizing Your Shadow Messages (Shadow Message Workshop, Part II)

Alchemy is a power or process that profoundly transforms something into a new and better version of itself. Over the centuries, alchemy was used in a physical sense to attempt to transmute impure or base metals like lead into superior and purer metals like gold. The word *alchemizing* is also used in relation to the human psyche and in personal development.

By alchemizing thoughts, behaviors, and beliefs that no longer serve us into something profoundly more helpful, we are empowered to create more autonomy over our lives. In this exercise, we will confront those agents of resistance—our Shadow Messages—and use the magic of alchemy to transmute them into helpful Supportive Statements that reinforce our growth and success.

Before you can alchemize your Shadow Messages, you'll first need to identify them, so if you haven't already done so, turn back to the exercise "Identifying Your Shadow Messages," also known as Part I of the Shadow Messages workshop, and complete that before continuing.

Now that you've spent some time identifying your Shadow Messages, it is time to look those scary little guys in the eye and do something wild and counterintuitive—invite them in for tea and a conversation. Follow the steps below to begin.

1. Review your Shadow Messages from Part I of the Shadow Messages Workshop, "Identifying Your Shadow Messages," and select one of your Shadow Messages to explore.

2. Choose three of the journal prompts listed on the next page.

3. Journal about your Shadow Message by using the journal prompts. Write as much as you can, and approach this with curiosity. You may want to imagine your Shadow Message as a child. Feel free to ask it questions, and write down what messages you imagine it is trying to tell you.

Journal Prompts

- How is this Shadow Message keeping me too comfortable or stuck?
- How does this Shadow Message benefit me?
- In what ways does this Shadow Message feel constrictive?
- What are the best and worst things that could happen if this Shadow Message is true?
- What could happen if the opposite of this Shadow Message is true?
- Write about a situation in the past when a similar Shadow Message came up.
- If my Shadow Message were a character, what would they be like?
- Write about a time when I overcame a limitation belief or fear.
- What would a brave person do if confronted with this limitation?
- What will happen if I never move forward with my desire?
- What will happen if I do move forward with my desire despite the Shadow Message?
- If this Shadow Message were a villain, how could I be the hero?
- If the Shadow Message were a lie, what would be the truth?

- How would my future self move past this limitation?
- What could be on the other side of my Shadow Message?
- Create a hilarious comedy sketch based on this Shadow Message.

Repeat this exercise for any additional Shadow Messages that you'd like to explore. Try choosing different journal prompts than before. It's okay to have fun with this. Feel free to get as creative as you'd like.

Well done on completing this exercise. By taking this time to reflect, you have shown your courage and willingness to be open to positive change. Not everyone is willing to do the inner work it takes to create the stability and strength to overcome sabotaging thoughts. You are worthy of achieving your desires, and by exploring your Shadow Messages, you've just taken a *huge* leap in the direction of manifesting them!

Now that you've taken time to explore what some of your Shadow Messages have to say, you have the opportunity to alchemize them into Supportive Statements. As we learned earlier in this chapter, it is possible to imprint our subconscious mind with new, better thoughts and beliefs. By going through the process of examining your Shadow Messages and then replacing them with upgraded, positive internal statements, you can move into alignment with the desires you wish to manifest.

When you imagine your dream life, chances are you envision a version of yourself who is a little different from who you are now. Perhaps future you is more confident, more resilient, and able to carve out time for her needs. Perhaps she is fully able to receive love and support from others without feeling discomfort. She feels in control of life and is respected and appreciated.

She lives a life of wellness and does the things that make her truly happy. How do we bridge the gap between who we are now and who we need to become in order to be a receptacle for our greatest manifestations? We start becoming her *now*.

Does future you worry about what outfit to wear to workouts? Does she lose sleep over a guy she's never met who didn't text her? Does future you fear what Tina from Accounting will think if she stumbles across your YouTube page? I don't think so. I think future you has much more important things to occupy her precious life-force energy—like living an awesome life.

Let's go ahead and alchemize those Shadow Messages into more positive statements that will support your mindset in becoming the person you need to be to begin attracting your desires into your life, starting now.

This is a four-step process, and good news—if you've already completed the "Identifying Your Shadow Messages" exercise in the first part of the Shadow Message Workshop, then you're familiar with how this will go and you probably have the first three steps already prepared. The fourth step is where the alchemizing magic happens.

Steps:

Desire: What is it you desire to manifest?
Action: What action could you take to help make it happen?
Shadow Messages: What Shadow Messages come up?
Supportive Statement: How could you take action but do it in a way that feels less scary? How could you love and support yourself in taking that action? What feels good about this action?

Let's revisit the three examples of the desires, actions, and Shadow Messages we used previously and add the fourth element, the Supportive Statement.

Example 1:

Desire: To feel healthier

Action: Spend one day a week going to a fitness class with my friend

Shadow Messages: What if I can't keep up with the rest of the class? What if everyone there is super fit and I look like the odd one out? What if I bump into someone from work when I'm all sweaty?

Supportive Statement: I will attend a class, and I will also prepare beforehand so that I know what to expect and can feel a little more confident about jumping into something brand-new. I will ask my friend what kind of clothing and equipment I'll need so I'll feel prepared before I arrive. I expect to feel some discomfort since this workout will be new to me. I'm choosing to be brave and not judge myself as I experience this new class. It is okay with me if I can't keep up with everyone else's level of fitness in the first class. I'm excited to try this class! It could be a whole new enjoyable experience for me and bring me amazing health benefits as well. I feel grateful that I will have a friend there with me.

Example 2:

Desire: To follow my passion

Action: Start a social media channel on a topic I'm passionate about

Shadow Messages: What if I don't get many followers? The proper equipment is probably too expensive. What if my parents/my ex/someone from work sees it? What if people leave negative comments?

Supportive Statement: I choose to be brave. My soul does not want to hide anymore. I don't want to feel unworthy. I see others experiencing so much joy and influence online as they share their message. I have a message and passions to share with likeminded people, so I am choosing to step past my insecurities and start small by creating a handful of posts and seeing how that feels to me. I reserve the right to change direction at any time. I refuse to feel stuck; I want to be in creative flow and share inspiration as it comes to me. I can use the equipment I already have. I release control of having to know or map out the full plan. I will just have fun taking the first thrilling steps!

Example 3:

Desire: To find love
Action: Go on a dating site and be open to going on dates
Shadow Messages: At my age, there are no great partners left. Dating sites are so cringe; it feels like I'm desperate. What if I get catfished by someone with a fake profile? What if I like someone and they end up ghosting me? What if I land a date but then they stand me up?
Supportive Statement: My heart's desire to have a loving, long-term partnership is much deeper and stronger than the limiting thoughts about what could go wrong. I am curious about online dating, but I also want to respect my need for safety. I will take my time to research which sites I feel comfortable with because they allow me the control to feel safe when interacting with potential dates. I am creating a love list of my desired traits in a partner so I can have clarity in knowing what I desire without feeling lost or swept up in the process. I will seek out dating and relationship advice from blogs and books to help me navigate this journey. I expect to feel first-date nerves, and that's okay with me; it's completely natural. Along with dating, I will also be taking some self-love and self-care actions to help me feel confident and elevate my vibration. I'm excited, ready, and open to meeting the right match for me.

Now it's your turn! Grab your journal and begin alchemizing your Shadow Messages into Supportive Statements. If you get stuck on scary Shadow Messages, try confronting them with this Magic Manifester Statement:

> Thank you for your message. I hear you, and I understand your concerns. You have kept me safe, but I'm a full-grown adult and I know what I'm doing. I'm intentionally expanding my life, and I'm going to be stretching past some of these limitations to attract greater things and live a life that feels more expansive to my heart and soul.

Once you've created your Supportive Statements, read them often. You might like to keep them next to your bed to read upon awaking and just before falling asleep, as you would with mantras and affirmations. In this way you can begin to imprint these new, positive thoughts in your mind so they become a natural part of your mindset.

Congratulations on completing the Shadow Messages Workshop! Use the tools you've learned to alchemize any scary or self-sabotaging messages that come up during your manifesting journey.

Envisioning the Future You

Think about the heart and soul desires that you'd most like to manifest and imagine *who* you will become when these desires come to fruition in your life. Imagine how you will move, act, feel, look, sound, behave, respond to others, share with others. Connect energetically with the future you who has all her heart and soul desires manifested. Does she feel happier? Freer? Lighter? More able to share her inner light with others? Take a moment to imagine this future you who is living her best life and manifesting her desires with ease.

In this exercise, you'll create a sensory tool to help you connect with the future version of yourself and inspire you to bring her essence into your present life. Choose the tool you'd like to create from the suggestions below. Or, you might think of other ways to envision the new you. It's up to you. Just have fun creating!

Vision Board

Use a poster board, scissors, glue, and images cut from magazines to create a collage of the things you'd like to manifest in your life. Incorporate words that will describe the essence of the future you who lives in a world where her desires have manifested. Find images that portray how she feels. Use colors to communicate a mood of calmness, excitement, or other desired emotions. When you're finished, display your board in a place where you will see it often.

Digital Vision Board

Create a digital vision board to keep as a file on your computer or device or to use as a screen saver. You can use free graphic design tools such as Canva to make an inspirational digital collage in the size of your choice and then add images that align with your desires. Alternatively, you could create a private Pinterest board to collect images and ideas that align with the way you want to live once your desires are manifested. You can view your digital vision board daily to connect with the essence of the future you.

Movie Screen Visualization

This is an eyes-closed meditation that works well as you drift off to sleep. Using the power of your mind, visualize a movie screen in front of you and imagine a day in the life of the future version of you—the you who lives a great life and is able to manifest her desires with ease. Where does she live? What is her morning routine? What activities does she do during the day? Who does she spend time with? What does she eat for dinner? What music is playing in the background? Follow her journey over the course of an imaginary day and feel all the good emotions that arise as you watch her experiencing a day in her life. Do this nightly or as often as you wish, following her journey and enhancing it along the way. Does she travel to different destinations every night? To make this a sensory experience, choose a small object in your house that sparks joy. It could be a crystal, a piece of jewelry, a beloved trinket, or a book. When you visualize your future self on the movie screen at night, imagine that she has that object with her. See it in her home or see her wearing it. Allow this object to become a visual reminder of the desires you wish to manifest and imagine that it holds an energetic link between your present self and your future self.

Future-You Wish List

This can be done using a physical journal or a notes app on your phone or computer. Create a wish list for your future self. You might like to include travel destinations, activities to try, topics to research, items to purchase, books to read, courses to take, events to attend, people to network with, guests to invite to a dinner party, projects to launch, and more. Remember, this is a wish list, so it doesn't have to be realistic. Let your imagination flow. Revisit your wish list regularly.

Future-You Playlist

When you imagine your future, what emotions do you desire to feel in that life? Create a playlist of songs that will act as a backdrop to your most amazing life. Does it start with upbeat music to dance to and then transform into more of a chill vibe? What songs mirror the mood you intend to set and the emotion you desire to feel? Explore your favorite music app, and once you've curated your playlist, use it to remind yourself of the good feelings you wish to attract into your life, starting today.

Scripting

Imagine your dream life has already come true and begin writing about it in the present tense, as though you're living it right now. Describe every detail—what your day looks like, how you feel, who you're with, and even the sounds, sights, and smells around you. Focus on the emotions and gratitude you experience in this new reality. Let your imagination flow freely. Repeat this exercise as often as you like (perhaps with each new moon) to strengthen your connection to your vision.

The Energy Awareness Challenge

I once lived in a neighborhood where the local traffic became truly chaotic around rush hour. The streets were jammed up with cars, no one wanted to let anybody into their lane, they were honking their horns, and impatient pedestrians were darting out in front of traffic. It had me all stressed out, every day, twice a day. I did not look forward to driving anywhere in the early evening because it was just so annoying and brought my whole vibe down.

One day I decided that it just wasn't worth getting so stressed about. I came up with an idea to do "30 Days of Zen." I challenged myself to not get stressed out by traffic, or anything else, for 30 days. I wanted to see if this would shift my reality—and it did. I employed a variety of techniques to avoid feeling stressed.

I listened to uplifting music in my car and even added a warming massage pad to my seat to enjoy while waiting around in traffic. After a few days, it seemed that the blocked streets weren't as bad as I had once experienced them, and feeling less stressed in traffic meant I was less stressed in my work life and with friends and family.

This was really an experiment in letting go. Where once I felt I had to maintain control over everything around me, I experimented for 30 days with just not doing that. My work life became less pressured and more enjoyable, and I didn't get caught up in other people's drama. Life started to up-level. These external improvements reflected my internal shift. As I look back now, I can see that by not becoming distracted by external influences I wasn't aligned with, my focus and precious life-force energy were reserved for the things that truly enhanced my lifestyle.

It's important for us to become aware of where our energy is getting drained or strained and to address it as best we can. A simple decision to keep returning to a state of Zen or a high vibration can be all that's needed to lift ourselves out of stress and experience more harmony. Of course, there are some stressors that can't be avoided. But we can challenge ourselves to keep returning to a more peaceful state as many times as it takes. Small internal choices like this can result in external shifts that might surprise you.

Your Energy Awareness Challenge for the remainder of this cycle (approximately one month) is to keep returning to good-feeling energy as often as possible. Follow the steps below to help yourself do this.

1. In a journal you keep next to your bed, make a list of your heart and soul desires (from the Heart and Soul Desires Meditation activity earlier in this chapter).

2. Each morning upon awaking, review your list of heart and soul desires. Imagine how you will feel when they come into manifestation. You may feel happy, empowered, relaxed, confident, at ease. Whatever it is, feel those feelings fully and enjoy them for a few moments.

3. Choose one word that sums up your feelings. This is your good-feeling word.

4. Assign a color to this good feeling that you are experiencing.

5. Now imagine that you are inside a giant invisible bubble that extends a few feet from you in all directions. Picture this imaginary bubble filling up with your good-feeling color.

6. In your mind or aloud, say your good-feeling word. This will help you connect to the essence of your energy bubble.

7. Take this energy bubble with you during this cycle. Practice returning to it several times a day by simply envisioning that it is there. You might be sitting at your office desk, or spending time with people you love, or running errands. Whatever you are doing throughout

the day, imagine yourself inside your good-feeling bubble as much as possible.

8. If a distraction or stressor occurs and you forget about your bubble, return to it as soon as you remember it. Keep returning to it each morning and whenever you can during each day of your current cycle.

9. Use your good-feeling word while imagining the color of your energy bubble to help you return to it.

10. At the end of your cycle, journal about the experience of being inside your energy bubble and any insights that this practice brought you.

Earthing

During the Attune phase, we may not feel like taking part in high-energy workouts or strenuous activities, so this could be the perfect time to get outdoors and into nature. *Earthing*, also known as *grounding*, is the practice of walking barefoot on the soil or the sand or swimming in a body of water. When we do this, we come into direct contact with the low-level magnetic field and energetic pulsations of the Earth that can support stress reduction and healing.[6] It is believed that the Earth's free (or mobile) electrons pass around and into our body through the body's energetic points and meridians. Earthing has been shown to reduce inflammation, help with sleep, reduce pain, relax the nervous system, and improve circulation, among many other benefits.

Being in nature, earthing, and breathing fresh outdoor air also improve the health of our gut microbiome, which can lead to a stronger immune system.[7] According to physician Zach Bush, we are a reflection of the diversity in nature, and we can turn to the natural world to help us diversify our microbiome in order to improve our health. He believes the ecosystem has healing potential. When we eat unprocessed, whole foods, touch nature—the soil, sand, or within a body of water—and breathe in real ecosystems, we will be in symbiosis with the earth and improve our immune system and adaptability. Visiting a variety of ecosystems can help to create more biodiversity in your body's microbiome.

My weekly walks by the ocean have diversified into excursions on various hiking trails, including a redwood grove where I once explored for an hour, breathing in the natural aromatics and touching the bark and leaves of the trees.

Exercise:

During the Attune phase, try incorporating gentle movement and stretching, walking, hiking, or yoga in a place with lots of trees and plants. You could also prepare a simple picnic or lie in a patch of sun for 15 minutes or more with your bare feet touching the earth.

Honing Your Intuition

Waiting for answers from the outside world? Now is the best time to practice going within for the answer. When you create quiet time to be still, you can tap in to your inner knowing, a quiet voice or feeling that guides you in decisions and perceptions without relying on logical reasoning. Tuning in to your authentic inner voice and listening for the next small step can help you traverse the unknown. The logical mind overflows with questions and judgments and can keep us stuck in indecision for years. There are times when the logical mind is essential, but there are also times when it can get in our way. Practice becoming familiar with the subtle nudge that tells you to take a chance, trust an insight, follow a passion, or change course, even when you can't fully explain why. Intuition taps into patterns and insights gathered from experiences, emotions, and our subconscious mind, allowing us to sense connections and possibilities beyond conscious awareness. It's a skill that grows sharper when we pay attention to it and honor its presence in our lives. Intuition can also feel like a deeply personal and spiritual tool, connecting us to something greater than ourselves. Hone your intuition by creating spaces of calm, creativity, and openness. Honoring your inner voice and balancing logic with instinct can lead you toward decisions that feel authentic and aligned with your highest good. ntuition is your inner compass, always available to guide you when you cultivate the quiet awareness to receive its messages. If you're struggling to make a decision, try flipping a coin. Assign heads to one option and tails to the other. Once the coin lands, pause and notce your immediate reaction. Do you feel happy relief or disappointment about the result? That instinctive response is your inner guidance speaking. This simple exercise helps you tune in to your intuition and practice trust ng the wisdom within.

New Moon Activation

If you like the idea of a new moon ritual, use this short visualization and activation to invite the energy of the new moon to assist you in bringing your heart and soul desires into manifestation. You might want to set the scene with low lighting, soft music, candles, crystals, or anything else that feels aligned.

1. Take a moment to find a comfortable spot where you will not be disturbed for about 15 minutes. Take a few slow, deep breaths to center yourself and close your eyes.

2. Imagine the night sky. See the new moon appearing as a black circle, and as you gaze at it, notice just a tiny sliver of light along her edge, as this giant heavenly body slowly orbits to reveal a tiny crescent of light. The moon is just beginning her journey of reemerging into a new cycle.

3. Now imagine your heart and soul desires. Hold their energy in your hands and stretch your arms above your head and hold your hands up to the new moon. Release your desires to the new moon and watch in wonder as they float upward to merge with her. The thin white sliver of light will expand with each passing hour and day until reaching its potential at the full moon, lighting up your desires and expanding them.

4. Feel gratitude for the universal energies at play in your life. They are right there for you to tap into at any time. Your role is to take small steps toward making your desires real, and the Universe's role is to ignite them with cosmic energy. Imagine the powerful force of the moon doing her part to help bring them to fruition. The moon, a universal force that affects the tides and our bodies, sends us all her energetic influence, and we can begin to feel trust in the Universe and cosmic cycles, knowing that they are forever moving things along. Imagine that you no longer have to push things forward alone.

5. Repeat this new moon activation: *I am worthy of receiving my heart and soul desires. I align with the*

natural energies of the Universe to assist me in bringing my desires into manifestation for the highest good of all. Thank you, thank you, thank you. And so it is.

6. Align with the natural, powerful energetic cycles of creation and visualize your heart and soul desires manifesting. You are in partnership with the Universe! Take a few minutes to visualize your heart and soul desires and watch them coming into manifestation before your eyes.

7. Take a few deep, cleansing breaths and slowly wiggle your fingers and toes. When you're ready, open your eyes.

Divine Downloads

Has the Universe taught you yet that you can't do everything yourself? And come to think of it, why would you want to? Support is available. When we discover the magic of cycles, we decide that we actually *don't* want to do everything ourselves; instead, we want to rest sometimes, and we want to have fun too. We learn that there are bigger forces of energy at play, and we can turn to a higher source to offer us support and inspiration.

If you're a believer, as I am, in a Divine universal energy of creation—whether you call this God, the Creator, Source energy, the Universe, or something else—then you may have a practice of communing with or even co-creating with this higher power. Whether you pray, meditate, chant, or connect through sacred texts or rituals, you may have felt this presence or guiding influence in your life.

As a small child I was taken to church by my parents to attend Sunday school while they attended the Christian service in the church. At Sunday school we learned that God was an all-knowing bearded man in Heaven who sat on a golden throne atop a cloud and could see everything that happened on the Earth. We learned not to sin, and that we should ask for forgiveness for any wrongdoings. By the time I was in high school, our family had stopped going to church, but I was left with that same impression of who or what God was until I delved deeper into spirituality in my 20s.

Although my adult mind could better understand the concept of a universal force of creation and the benefits of connecting with this force, I found it difficult to get past the image I had of God as a bearded man sitting on a throne in the sky. My friends who also studied and practiced spirituality would talk about how they would "have conversations" with God and had opened up a dialogue and "friendship with the Creator." Whenever I tried to do this I felt as if I was approaching a very busy and judgmental king on a throne and hesitantly pulling at his robe to ask him a silly question. Didn't he have much more important things to do in the world than to help me find a boyfriend, navigate the latest office drama, or heal my stress headache? My attempts to pray felt like an interruption of the Almighty's time, and that my desires, requests, and problems were small fry compared to the other worldly problems he was dealing with.

This was such a huge block for me, and all the while every spiritual teaching I was learning emphasized the importance of having a relationship with the Creator. When I tried to imagine the Creator as just a neutral energy, neither male nor female, I felt like I was talking to a computer and I just couldn't connect, try as I might. Finally, I decided to do something revolutionary—something that felt a little wrong and that I kept secret. I started to connect with the *feminine* aspect of God. I'm not talking about any particular angel or goddess, I'm talking about the Divine feminine expression of the Creator, also known as the Shechinah. This allowed my breakthrough, and I started to feel at ease and comfortable with "having conversations" with this Divine Mother energy. It acted as a conduit in forming a daily connection with the energy of the Creator. Today, I can speak to the Creator as a Divine force and not get hung up on whether it is male or female. I now view the Creator as a unifying force that contains both male and female aspects.

Co-creating with this energy of the Divine as my partner is my favorite thing in the world. I am happy that I persisted in trying to connect with this Source, and that I now feel a closeness to and reverence for this force in my life. When I consider all that I have manifested over the past few years, I view each gift, blessing, and accomplishment as a result of co-creation with this benevolent force that holds a power far greater than my limited capabilities. I believe that we each have the ability to invite in and receive Divine inspiration directly from the Universe, God, Source, the Creator—and I call these Divine Downloads.

I have set out a few exercises to explore so you can invite this energy into your life, or try new ways to enhance it. You can practice tuning in to receive inspiration regularly, not just during the Attune phase. "What does it feel like to receive a Divine Downland?" you might ask. What I have found is that Divine Downloads are often not linear, but they feel good and light you up. You may receive big-picture flashes and visions of future inspiration, or, more often than not, just an inkling or clue that unfolds in front of you one small step at a time. It can feel like following a trail of clues, and once you see the big picture unfold, it is quite magical. At first this path felt counterintuitive, as I am a planner by nature—someone who needs to know what will be happening six months from now so I can prepare. It has really been a leap of faith to follow the breadcrumbs of my Divine Downloads and build trust in the Creator's loving guidance and delightful surprises. This magic is available to all of us, but to receive Divine Downloads, you need to create space for them. During the Attune phase, embrace rest, stillness, and spaciousness to allow space to tune in, listen, ask, imagine, and receive. Here are some ways to do this, but perhaps you can think of even more.

- Create a Universe to-do list. Start a page in your journal with the heading "Universe To-Do List" and freely list anything you need support on. This might include finding the right person for something you need help with, calling in the right systems to help you manifest a desire, or attracting the resources you need for a passion project. Be open to clues that might come up during this cycle.

- Take intentional space and time in your schedule to just "be" and rest. Choose a time and space where you won't be disturbed and consciously ask to receive insight, love, direction, and support. Journal your thoughts and feelings.

- Inspiration can pop up when we engage in repetitive actions. Washing dishes, doing makeup, cleaning, or folding laundry are all examples of this. We often go into exploratory thinking, daydreaming, and problem-solving when we are doing things that don't require a lot of active attention. In these times we can more easily access the unlimited creative realm. Pose a question or problem to solve to yourself before you undertake these daily tasks. If you do not receive a message, let it go; a Divine Download may be delivered to you a short time later.

- Set your journal and a pen beside your bed and pose a question to the Universe before you fall asleep. Write down whatever comes into your mind when you wake up in the morning.

- Visit a nature area, walk among the plants and trees, hear the birds and critters, breathe in the natural aromatics. Dwell in nature for a while and let your mind wander. Check in with yourself to see what your soul is craving, or if you are thinking of a particular person or a new approach to a project that spontaneously came up. If you don't have access to a forest or beach, a backyard or neighborhood garden could be your spot.

- Engage in creative projects by tapping into feminine energy. We all have both masculine and feminine energy to draw upon. Feminine energy is more about *being* than *doing*. Take time to lose yourself in drawing, coloring, crafting, painting, designing, dancing, or moving. Flow and connect to that wonderful feeling of high vibration to welcome in Divine Downloads, which may appear during your activity or shortly after.

- Follow your joy. This can appear counterintuitive, especially when there's so much to be done and so much that the logical mind is bringing to your attention. Reserve a few hours on a day when you don't have as many commitments and begin by asking yourself, *What is my soul craving to do today that's different from my usual schedule?* You may receive a feeling or an urge to catch up with a particular friend or to go to a particular location. Follow your inspiration and see what unfolds.

Becoming a Co-Creator

Through a partnership of co-creation with a power greater than ourselves—whether you experience this as the Universe, Source energy, God, the Creator, Archangels, or something else—I believe we all do have the power to bring our most cherished heart and soul desires into manifestation. In my studies of ancient spiritual practices, a Kabbalah teacher once shared a simple yet profound story with me. Among the many parables of mighty biblical Matriarchs, Patriarchs, spiritual luminaries, and sages, this one stuck in my memory because it involved a tiny mouse and an elephant. As the story goes, a mouse was playing in a field and having fun kicking up lots of dust as he circled around in the dirt. Soon an elephant sauntered along and inquired as to what the mouse was doing. "Look at all these dust clouds I'm making," the mouse said. The elephant smiled and gently placed his trunk in front of the mouse and invited him to scamper up his trunk and onto his back. The mouse hopped aboard the elephant's back, enjoying the view from such a lofty height, and the elephant began to walk across the field. "Wow!" the mouse exclaimed "Now look at all the *huge* dust clouds I'm making from up here!" I'm pretty sure at this point the elephant winked. Or not. But it feels right. The message is simple—when we co-create with a power greater than us, it generates a much more satisfying impact. I've found that by cultivating a daily practice of connecting to a higher source through meditation or prayer, my life has benefited in countless ways. It's also a reminder for us not to lose appreciation for our connection with a higher power, or the universal energies that ignite the orbits of the planets, no less. We don't have to constantly push and exert physical effort to bring our desires into manifestation. We can leverage the gigantic power of universal energies.

· ·

Lifestyle Attunement

Enjoy exploring these lifestyle-enhancing ideas during your Attune phase.

Mind

- Keep your schedule light and say no to unnecessary commitments during this phase.
- Take technology breaks when possible.
- Try not to schedule projects that require long periods of focus.
- This is a time to delegate what responsibilities you can.
- Consider blocking out time for rest and reflection. When we relax and quiet our mind, brilliant ideas can flow to us.
- While you meditate, diffuse essential oils with purifying and protective qualities, such as lemon and frankincense.
- Try space clearing prior to meditating by using a sound bowl or by burning sage or palo santo.
- Use low lighting or mood lighting to create a restful vibe.
- Play healing-frequency music or binaural beats to support relaxation.
- Create a manifestation bath ritual by adding your favorite aromatic salts or oils to warm bathwater and playing some meditative music while envisioning your desires being manifested as you soak.

Body

- Skip intensive workouts during the Attune phase. Light and slow exercises such as stretching, gentle mat Pilates, walking, massaging your muscles with a foam roller, or yin yoga can be helpful in the afternoon or early evening.

- Sip coconut water to boost hydration.

- Consider foods that help with bloating and cravings if you are following your menstrual cycle, including antioxidant-rich colorful, non-starchy vegetables; omega-3-rich foods such as salmon and sardines; and citrus fruits for their high vitamin C content.

- Avoid a lot of sweet foods, as they can interfere with estrogen production. Legumes and low-glycemic fruits such as fresh apples and berries are a good choice.

- Winter-style dishes such as hearty soups and stews will feel nourishing in this phase.

- Prepare healthy comfort foods and ingredients prior to the Attune phase for low-key meal preparation while you rest.

- Practice good sleep hygiene. Create a sleep environment that is like a cave—cool, dark, and quiet.

- Consider wearing blue-light-filtering glasses when looking at screens after sunset to help your body naturally wind down for bedtime.

- Embrace lounging. Wear cozy, comfortable loungewear in soft or silky fabrics whenever possible.

- Nurture your skin with balms and oils. Apply them using self-massage movements to the feet and hands. Wear moisturizing foot creams under thick socks while you rest or sleep.
- For maximum hair growth, refrain from cutting it during this phase; wait until the next phase, Awaken.

Soul

- Pull oracle or tarot cards and do a reading.
- Be open to receiving Divine Downloads of intuition from higher sources. Take note of any intuitive inspirations or ideas in a journal or notes app.
- Learn about and connect with crystals. For example, clear quartz can be used to amplify your meditations.
- Connect with supportive energies or higher souls during prayer. Invite your higher guides, benevolent souls, or ancestors to join you in prayer and dedication.
- Consider starting a dream diary to capture your dreams.
- Repeat your personal mantras and other positive affirmations regularly.
- Before bed, write down any questions or support you'd like from the Universe. Upon awaking, use a notepad or journal to document your dreams and any messages you received.
- Research which astrological sign the moon is in and read about the energies available at this time.

Transitioning to the Next Phase

It may seem like you will never resurface from your comfy, cozy cocoon of the Attune phase, but as sure as the seedlings will start to push up through the dark Winter soil, you can trust that you too will emerge. Your energy will return and gain strength, along with ideas of actions to take to help move your desires forward into manifestation. As each phase of the cycle rolls into the next, we build a greater sense of trust in the Universe and in ourselves.

During the Attune phase you have deeply explored your most cherished desires and created powerful tools of affirmation to prime your mindset for receiving your manifestations. You have imprinted your subconscious mind (and continue to do so) with the beliefs that you are deserving of the life you desire and that it is within reach. You have felt the emotions of what it will feel like to manifest your dreams, and now you are ready to start embodying them.

In the Awaken phase, motivation and activity begin to rise and create their own momentum. Your heart and soul desires will start to take form right in front of your eyes. Taking forward-moving actions during the Awaken phase happens with ease since you will be leveraging the natural elevations of energy that occur during this phase. You will learn that there is a time for everything and that you don't have to feel pressured to fill your day with an impossible amount of tasks and activities. Scheduling your life will become fun as you create a holistic plan using the Cycle Habits Tracker and learn how to leverage your time by habit stacking and biohacking your way to wellness. Failing at habits will become a thing of the past. Magically, there will be time to do everything (just not all at once). You will gain a new level of success in adopting healthy habits that stick and help yourself move the needle in favor of your goals. The empowering phase of Awaken is ready when you are!

Chapter 5

AWAKEN

• • • • • • • • • •

> **Moon Phase:** Waxing Crescent, First Quarter, and Waxing Gibbous
> **Menstrual Phase:** Follicular (Preovulation)
> **Season:** Spring
> **Element:** Air
> **Energetic Attributes:** Intellect and Action
> **Essence:** Flirt, growth, arise, increase, develop, emerge, unfold, innovate, extend, launch, form, initiate, establish, commence, momentum, focus, movement, urge, influence

Shake off that dreamy Attune energy, it's time to Spring forward and take aligned action!

Tiny seedlings of possibility are bursting forth from the fertile soil and unfurling in the warm air. As they emerge, so do your vitality and ingenuity. Forward momentum takes hold, and it's ready to joyfully support you in bringing your dreams into reality.

When I first met Mia, a young mom of two preteen boys, we were mingling at a fundraising event in Newport Beach,

California. Like many of the women in attendance, Mia was fashionably dressed, had a fresh blowout, and looked gorgeously toned. As we chatted, it was no surprise to learn that she took morning Pilates classes—and that wasn't all she was fitting into her mornings. Mia's husband worked in finance and left the house early each morning, so she would get her two boys ready for school, drop them off, go to her Pilates class, run some errands, and then manage anything that needed to be done for a few out-of-state rental properties they owned. This all took place before her various lunch meetings, which, depending on the day, could be for any number of social networks, charitable event teams, or women's business associations. As she told me about her work with a local fundraising committee, a waiter drifted by and offered us some crispy cones filled with seared tuna and avocado. "No, thank you, I'm on a cleanse." Mia smiled tensely. We got to talking about nutrition and set up a coffee date for the following week.

When we met at the café, Mia shared with me that she'd been feeling a lot of pressure to keep up with her busy lifestyle. She confessed that by the early evenings, when her boys and husband came home, she was exhausted and they often ordered takeout. "I miss the days when I would cook healthy meals for the boys and try new recipes. My family loves my cooking!" Mia also felt that her body was changing, so she had cut calories and undertaken long hours of fasting, which contributed to a hormone imbalance. She would often binge on something sugary or drink diet sodas to "pep herself up." Mia felt like mood fluctuations were affecting her relationship because at times she couldn't help but snap at her husband. She showed me her sleep tracker to illustrate how she was "tired but wired" at the end of a long day and often had trouble sleeping. Most shocking of all, she confessed that she didn't even *like* her morning Pilates class, but she dragged herself there whether she felt like it or not.

Although Mia was very grateful for her beautiful life and family, she had been holding herself to impossible standards, and somewhere in the process of trying to be the perfect wife, mom, philanthropist, and businesswoman, she had lost her joy. When I asked Mia about the things that made her feel happy and healthy, she lit up and told me about going bike riding with her family around the bay and then stopping for a smoothie afterward. She also loved to take her boys stand-up paddleboarding, shopping for cool sneakers, and visiting nature conservation areas along the coast to learn about the local species. In Summer they loved to spend family days at the beach and swim in the ocean. "I love being near the water, maybe because I'm a Pisces?" Mia pondered. "Or maybe I was a mermaid in a past life?" she said with a childlike giggle. I began to see a playful side of Mia coming out—one that had long been sequestered by more pressing obligations.

It was clear that Mia was craving quality time with her family—wanting to nurture them with delicious meals, spend time with them in nature, and be fully present with them. She also longed for the freedom of having space in her schedule to just "be" and experience a deep sense of rest and rejuvenation. She wanted to cut down on restaurant meals and feed her body nutritious foods and feel good in her body without having to follow a punishing fitness and diet regimen.

As we sat together in the café, I told Mia about a system I had just designed to help women enjoy the healthy habits they love without feeling like a failure if they miss a day. It would also help them align their habits and activities to suit their hormonal phases so they didn't have to try to do everything all at once.

"Oh, that's what I need!" Mia said. She was ready to try a new way, since what she'd been doing hadn't been bringing her the health and happiness she deserved. I showed Mia the Cycle

Habits tracking system and we agreed to keep in touch and meet up again in a month.

The following month I was waiting in a busy juice bar for our follow-up session when Mia walked in and I was struck by how happy and relaxed she looked. Her hair flowed with a natural waviness and her skin had a sun-kissed glow. She was dressed comfortably and looked refreshed. Mia told me that she was going to meet the boys and her husband for a bike ride around the bay after our meeting.

"Wow, that's great you are finally going bike riding again," I said.

"Oh, we've been riding every Sunday. It's been great—and that's not all. . . ." She took out her iPad and showed me the screen. Her digital copy of the Cycle Habits Tracker was filled with colorful markings from her stylus pen to indicate the dates that she'd been doing her new healthy habits over the last month.

"Great job, Mia, I'm so happy for you! How do you feel?" I asked.

Mia began to tell me how she had changed her lifestyle. She'd let go of the commitments and classes that she was no longer interested in and delegated quite a few event tasks to other committee members who were more than happy to take them on. She no longer punished her body with restriction, and instead nurtured it with whole foods. Pointing to the Cycle Habits Tracker on her iPad, she said, "Look, I made twelve home-cooked meals last month. Can you believe it? That was something I had just written off as not doable before. *And* I took the boys out paddleboarding five times!"

Mia had also managed to fit in some self-care practices that reduced her stress, and she'd seen an improvement in her sleep. She'd done a great job of making a few shifts in her lifestyle that had already brought major benefits into her life. When I told Mia about the incredible changes I saw in her, she waved her iPad in the air and asked with a smile, "What kind of sorcery is this?"

Just as Mia did, you can create your *own* wellness magic. In the Awaken phase, you're going to learn how to get clear about your goals and create some healthy habits that you enjoy so you too can cycle into your best life ever.

During this phase we are future focused as we Awaken with vitality to journey forward with manifesting our dreams. The seeds of your heart and soul desires were planted in the fertile soil of the Attune phase and manifestation seedlings are now emerging. Feel the excitement of transmuting the metaphysical into the physical by aligning with the momentum of the Awaken phase.

Part of the menstrual cycle, the follicular phase begins as a woman finishes menstruation and lasts approximately 7 to 10 days. During this time the confidence-boosting hormone estrogen is on the rise, helping our body produce feel-good hormones like serotonin and dopamine, which make us better able to handle stress. In this Awaken phase, we are likely to feel an incremental boost in energy and have less of an appetite than at other times in our cycle, making this the perfect opportunity to begin adopting healthy habits. Whether it's moving our body in a fitness class or eating more nutritious whole foods to crowd out processed foods, we now have the energetic support available to help us pursue our wellness goals. As estrogen continues to increase throughout this phase, a woman's journey will eventually culminate in the main event of the menstrual cycle—ovulation, which we will talk more about in the next phase, Thrive. As we've discussed in previous chapters, each person's cycle is unique, so if you have irregular cycles or prefer not to align with your menstrual cycle, you may find it simpler to align with the moon cycle.

The consistent increase in estrogen in the menstrual cycle mirrors the expanding light of the moon that steadily grows night by night over the course of the waxing moon phase until she arrives at her peak ripeness as the full moon (which happens in the next phase, Thrive). As the moon's light gradually brightens, its gravitational and luminous effects subtly influence biological rhythms and growth patterns in various organisms.[1] The energy of growth abounds. Activity intensifies, and living systems align to support the emergence of new life.

The Awaken phase is aligned with the energy of Spring, which is energetically linked to the element of Air. As warm Spring air circulates, our spirits awaken and connection and communication are boosted. In spiritual traditions such as astrology and tarot, Air is symbolic of communication, intellect, and action. During the Awaken phase, our intellect can be sharp like a sword. Winds of change can blow through and effortlessly bring ideas to the next level of manifestation. Digital clouds can unify and interconnect us, upgrading the collective consciousness. Things can happen quickly. Seeds of possibility can suddenly begin to sprout and unfold before our eyes. Creativity can flow and innovative solutions can arise, so let's tap in to this uplifting energy.

We often "hope and wish" that our dreams will come true, and while there is a time for mindful metaphysical work (the Attune phase), that time has passed, and now we get to take an *active* role in our manifestation journey. We get to become co-creators with the Universe in shaping our destiny. The Awaken phase is not the time to energetically try to "will" our desires into manifestation, and it's not the time to let go of the dreams we feel we might be holding on to too tightly. This phase signals a time for aligned action.

In this forward-moving Awaken phase, we will want to ensure that our energy, attention, and focus are not distracted by unnecessary diversions. The more you focus on nurturing and building your intentions and goals without distraction during the Awaken phase, the more potent this time will be for you. As you travel along your Awaken journey, you will practice exercises to help you plan habits and goals, use this expansive energy to take quantum leaps into the future (where your dreams are already a reality), and become a clear channel for manifestation. You'll discover tools and techniques that heighten innovation as you create systems to support new realities so you can experience your manifestations' unfolding. There is plenty of space to play and be creative as you shape your desires into action steps and launch new initiatives. It's go time!

Where to Begin

There are two essential exercises that flow in sequence in this phase to help you begin manifesting your desires. They are followed by a section called "Awaken Phase Practices" that includes additional, optional practices and tools that you may also want to explore when you circle back to this phase in future cycles. The Awaken Phase Practices will support you as you return again and again to the Awaken phase and use the variety of tools offered to help facilitate your manifesting journey. They are not intended to be used all at once, but rather revisited in future cycles to keep things fun. However, if you have plenty of time set aside to explore the Awaken phase tools and exercises during your current cycle, then feel free to dive into as many of those additional practices as you'd like to. For your very first Awaken journey, start with these two core exercises:

1. Creative Brainstorming
2. Your Cycle Habits Journey

Set aside a minimum of 30 minutes for each exercise, and up to an hour, if possible. The duration of the entire Awaken phase might be anywhere from 7 to 12 days (depending on the length of your follicular phase, or your waxing moon alignment), and you can begin anytime within this time period.

If you have a natural menstrual cycle and are not currently on birth control, the best time to launch your Awaken phase exercises will be toward the end of menstruation. Day 1 of your cycle is the first day of menstruation (in the previous phase, Attune). You may start to feel the energies of the Awaken phase anywhere between approximately Day 3 and Day 6 of your cycle. When more naturally uplifting energy emerges, that's the indication to begin. If you're unsure and still experimenting with being more "in tune" with the energies of your cycle, then start around the time you finish menstruation, or before Day 6, if you can. Ideally, you will complete these exercises before ovulation (the Thrive phase), which typically begins about halfway through the menstrual cycle—around Day 14, approximately, if you have a 28-day cycle, but this can vary. If you are not already tracking your cycle, I recommend using an app or a wearable device to help you align with your menstrual cycle. View "Resources" on page 264 for suggestions.

If you are aligning your manifesting journey with the moon cycle, begin the Awaken phase exercises during the waxing crescent moon. To be more exact, if the new moon was Day 1 (part of the Attune phase), you could start your Awaken phase on from Day 3 to Day 6 of the moon phase. Try to start prior to the first quarter moon if you can. The goal is to finish your Awaken phase exercises before the full moon.

Do your best with timing, use your intuition, and please don't let the "when to begin" factor stress you out or derail your manifestation journey. This is *your* journey. The cycle will be here, ready for you, when you have the time to align with it, guaranteed. So if you are not able to do the recommended exercises during one cycle, try again next month. After all, you have countless attempts to try this, and lifetime access to natural energy cycles, so if you lose track, just hop back on when you're ready! As sure as the sun and moon continue to rise and set, the cycle will be here to support you, and each time you get a chance to align with it, you will become more and more familiar with its energies.

It's Time to Awaken!

You have arrived in the Spring time of your cycle. The Winter frost has melted away, and you can feel the warmth of the sun transferring its energy to you. The air is ripe with potential. It's time to take action and tend your seedlings of possibility.

1. Creative Brainstorming

Being active participants in manifesting our dreams entails setting the stage for our desires to flourish, coming up with supportive systems to help us achieve our goals with ease, and being open to inspiration on how we can align with our desires.

Whether it's love, abundance, wellness, a sense of purpose, connection, stability, freedom, passion for life, vitality, creativity, or something more that you want, notice that these ideals are all quite ethereal. You can't touch love. You can't go online and order up some stability, and although many have tried, you can't bottle wellness. These are ways of being. Modes of living. They are frequencies that you need to move into alignment with. The desires you want to manifest could stay up in the clouds forever—unless you find a way to tether them to the here and now.

So how do you transform the intangible into the tangible? How do you bring the invisible into physical existence? How do you acquire the immaterial? That's the kind of magic we'll be getting into during the Awaken phase. The merging of two worlds—the unmanifest and the manifest—begins now with this exercise so you can make your desires real and experience them in your life.

Approach this exercise in two parts. You could do both on the same day, or on different days during the Awaken phase. In this exercise you will unleash the full strength and capabilities of your mind. To do this, you have to separate your creative approach from your logical approach. Let's begin with the fun part first!

Part I: Creative

This is a creative space for expanding and building upon ideas with no limitations, and without getting into the logical mind (which is Part II of this activity). Follow the steps to get started.

1. Locate your list of desires from the Heart and Soul Desires Meditation from the previous phase, Attune. Write them on a fresh page in your journal.

2. Take a deep breath and set an intention that you want to access the part of your brain that supports creativity. You are going to put your "logical" mind on hold for now so you can channel a stream of uninterrupted creative ideas and write until you get them all out onto paper.

3. To access your creativity and playfulness, draw a small, simple picture. It could be of an animal, a landscape, a cartoon. If you can't think of anything to draw, look

around and draw something that you see—maybe an object on your desk, or something outside the window. Spend up to five minutes on your drawing.

4. Choose one of your Heart and Soul Desires to begin with and ask the following question: *How can I bring this desire to life?*

5. Write down *all* of your ideas, even the crazy ones, without stopping to think about them. Just keep writing idea after idea like a stream of water. Challenge yourself to see how many ideas you can write in the next few minutes. Keep the ideas coming, keep flowing, do not stop. Write until all the ideas are laid out on paper.

6. Repeat this process for any additional desires.

Example:

Desire: To live abundantly

Ideas: Talk to my neighbor about tutoring his son, create an ebook or online course, make money from my hobbies, sell jewelry, ask my friend Mel to help me make a website, research online-income ideas, reread that book about money, partner with my friend to sell products, open a market stall, sell my services to local businesses, teach corporate employees skills, host an event in my town, put flyers in the coffee shop to promote my idea, sell my crafts online, look into drop-shipping product ideas, ask my colleague about that side business he mentioned, create an online workshop, start a social media channel, research trending products, promote products on social media, do a TED Talk about a topic, do keynote speaking and get an agent, help a local business with online marketing, offer bookkeeping as a service, start a blog, be a virtual assistant once a week, design graphics, offer yoga classes locally, teach online, learn a new skill, get crowdfunding for my idea, create a how-to guide.

Part II: Logical

After all your creative ideas are captured on paper, you can turn to your analytical mind to review them in a logical way. This is the time to allocate some ideas to the back burner and decide which ones to take forward in this cycle. Follow the steps to begin.

1. Select one of the desires you worked on in Part I of this Creative Brainstorm and look over the ideas you generated.
2. Circle your favorite ideas. Choose at least five.
3. Take one of your ideas and journal on these questions:

    What resources do I need to start this?

    How can I make time for this?

    What would it take to bring this idea to life?

    What small steps can I take this week to get started?

    What is the first step?

    Repeat this for any additional ideas you'd like to explore.

4. Review your notes from Step 3 and create two categories, Actions and Habits. Actions are one-off things you can add to a task list or schedule in your calendar to kick off your goals (e.g., research a topic, make a call, sign up for a course). Habits are things you'd like to do *regularly* or consistently over the course of a month (e.g., work out,

meditate, review your budget, get some sun). Keep hold of the Habits; we'll be using them in the next exercise.

Great job! You are doing magical work here to bring your desires into manifestation. Now you have some real-life actions to initiate and habits to take forward, but don't be overwhelmed. We're going to incorporate them in a way that aligns with your *energy* (not your time), and it's going to be a flexible system that lets you feel in control and supported.

2. Your Cycle Habits Journey

It's time to leverage this action-oriented Awaken energy and create some habits and supportive systems that will pave the way for your future manifestations. How do you feel when you hear the word *habits*? Perhaps you've tried to establish new habits or resolutions in the past, but they've fallen off your schedule at some point? Does the thought of creating habits give you a twinge of anxiety? We all know it's healthy to stretch our comfort zone now and then to create positive change, but past disappointments over failed habit-keeping can create a roadblock on our manifesting journey. There is good news, though: I created a solution that I think you'll love! It's time to embrace Cycle Habits.

Cycle Habits are tracked over the course of a month (not a day), because who feels like doing a high intensity fitness class when you're in rest mode or menstruating? The burden of trying to keep up with daily habits can create unnecessary stress or guilt and often leads to burnout, especially for perfectionists like me. When we read about daily habits, it sounds logical— incorporating things that will point us in the direction of our goals each and every day. But in reality it creates pressure from the time we wake up until the time we go to sleep to check off the items on our list of habits. The unrealistic crunch of daily habits for women can also result in the abandonment of certain habits altogether, many of which may be perfectly healthy to continue with *on rotation* in our schedule, but not daily.

Daily Habits Are Not Designed for Women

Daily habit tracking is a one-size-fits-all approach that doesn't account for the unique needs and rhythms of women's bodies. From hormonal fluctuations throughout the menstrual cycle to the different ways women experience energy, stress, and well-being than men, typical habit frameworks fail to honor these natural variations. As a result, many women struggle to maintain consistency in generic routines, feeling disconnected or frustrated by approaches that don't align with their physical and emotional states. *What about all the research that shows the amazing benefits of keeping up with daily habits?* you might be wondering. Most of the research cited in studies and books about the benefits of daily habits was conducted on men. Unfortunately, there is a gender bias in medical research, and females remain underrepresented even today.[2] This is slowly changing, but it's something to keep in mind when we read or hear about studies on health, habit forming, fitness, and more. There's a huge difference between the inherent energies, biologies, and hormones of men and women. Men are on a daily rhythm, receiving secretions of the powerhouse hormone testosterone each day (more in the morning, tapering off at night),[3] whereas women are on a fluctuating hormonal cycle that is closer to a monthly rhythm, and we receive a spike of testosterone (much less than men do) once per cycle around ovulation (the Thrive phase). While most days follow the same predictable energetic rhythms for men, for women, each day is different due to the constant fluctuations of our hormones. It's only when we view them over the course of a month that we can see a predictable pattern to use in leveraging our cycles of energy. This is why I felt called to develop the Cycle Habits system specifically for women. I've learned to adopt a monthly habit-tracking schedule that has built-in flexibility so I can feel good about aligning my lifestyle with my menstrual cycle or the moon cycle. While *daily* habits are not realistic, there are still huge gains to be made by repeating habits *regularly* over the course of a month.

So, what are Cycle Habits? They are small, repeatable habits that have a compounding effect on the direction of your life. Imagine you are the navigator on a ship. By shifting the navigation by just one degree, you can eventually arrive at a destination thousands of miles from your original course. This is the power of small habits done consistently. When it comes to habits that optimize our wellness, we're either doing them, or we're not. There's not a *between* for gaining the kind of compounding benefits that healthy habits can yield, so let's dive in and create just a few that can be realistically incorporated over the course of a month, and then build from there.

The trick is to list all the habits you'd like to do for each phase (Attune, Awaken, Thrive, and Surrender) and track them over the course of one menstrual or moon cycle. Refer to the Cycle Magic chart and phase summaries in Chapter 3 to review the predominant energies of each phase. I suggest beginning with three to five habits in total and adding more as you become familiar with the process. What does this look like in action?

Introducing Your Cycle Habits Tracker

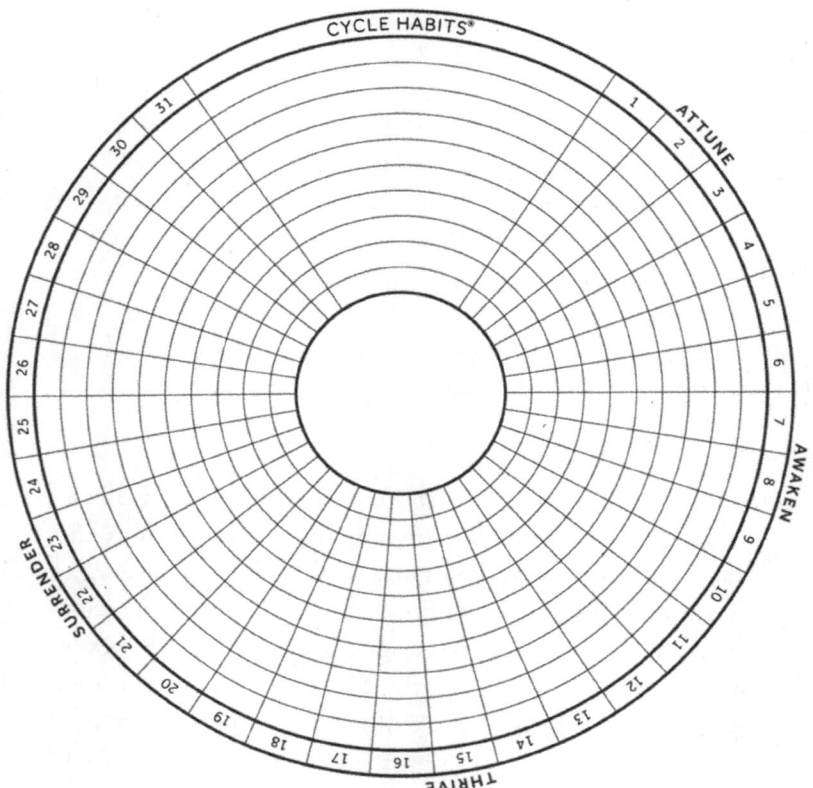

Your Cycle Habits Tracker may look something like this after one cycle of tracking habits:

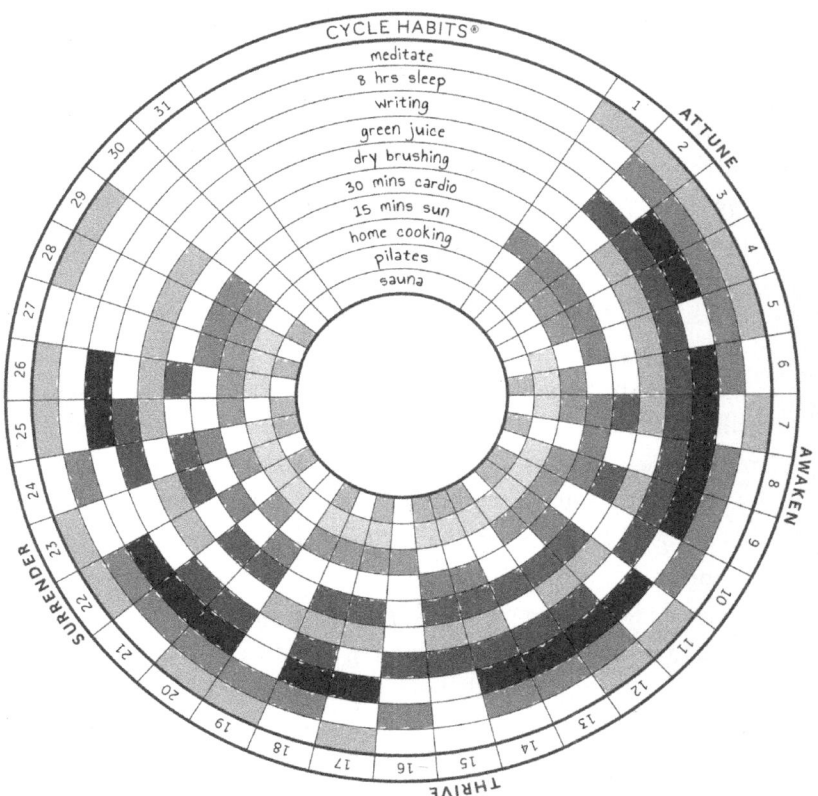

Notice how during this month I did certain habits more in certain phases? For example, I meditated almost every day during the Attune phase—which is the time for rest and contemplation. I did more cardio during the Thrive phase, the time for action and energy. The more you track, the more you will begin to understand how your habits can be streamlined with your cycle for a more aligned life and better outcomes for your overall wellness.

For now, you can just list the habits you want to initiate in this Awaken phase if you'd like to keep it simple to begin with. The Cycle Habits Tracker system allows for the flexibility of engaging in certain habits during certain phases without feeling like a failure if you don't keep up with them daily. The pressure of performing a list of nonnegotiable daily habits can feel like you're on a hamster wheel. Where is the joy in that? Of course, some habits may be easy and joyful to stick to daily, such as waking up to a large glass of water with lemon on most days or doing some light stretching. But when it comes to exercise, dietary habits, and self-care, these habits will likely fluctuate depending on the phase you're in.

Even if you're not engaging in certain habits daily, you can still achieve success by keeping them in your rotation long-term to reap their benefits in your life. Cycle Habits also allows for variety throughout the month, so that you are not in a position of having to cram too many habits into a daily regimen and then failing or feeling overwhelmed.

Cycle Habits are powerful steps in the direction of the up-leveled future you envision. Aligning your lifestyle habits with your cycle is likely to work much better for you than using the typical way our society packages time—in days, workweeks, weekends, and so on. So while we do acknowledge the power and compound effect of performing daily habits, we don't get stuck on the *daily* part of it. Sometimes you may decide to skip some or all of your habits for a day or two to rest or as you enjoy a fun life celebration or trip, and that's a good thing. You have the freedom to adjust, tweak, and return to your Cycle Habits to get right back to it. When you start experiencing the compound results and flexibility of your Cycle Habits, I promise, you will be hooked!

Now it's your turn. Grab your journal and start listing some Cycle Habits you'd like to try out. Or, if you completed the

Creative Brainstorming exercise, you already have some habits to consider.

Use the Cycle Habits Tracker to keep yourself inspired and on course. Visit cyclehabits.com/tracker to download your blank Cycle Habits Tracker sheet. Print as many copies as you like, or use the Cycle Habits Tracker digitally by opening the file you downloaded with a PDF annotation app such as Goodnotes or Canva on your tablet, phone, or desktop.

Enter your top 10 (or fewer) habits for the month into the Cycle Habits Tracker and keep track of your habits by filling in the corresponding spaces as you make your way around your cycle, whether it's your menstrual cycle or the moon cycle. Happy cycling!

The Awakened Brain

As your estrogen level rises during the follicular phase, something incredible happens in the brain—it becomes primed for creativity, motivation, and new ideas, making it the perfect time to transform dreams into reality. Elevated estrogen stimulates the production of brain-derived neurotrophic factor (BDNF), enhancing cognitive flexibility and neuroplasticity, the brain's capacity to form new neural connections through learning, memory, and adaptation.[4] This surge supports the development of new habits, skills, and thought patterns, creating fertile ground for creativity, innovative thinking, and problem-solving. It also enhances the prefrontal cortex's functionality, boosting planning, decision-making, and attention. These changes make it easier to set goals, focus intentions, and visualize outcomes vividly, creating fertile ground for personal growth and transformation. An elevated estrogen level also regulates mood by increasing serotonin and dopamine production, which fosters positivity and persistence.[5] Dopamine sensitivity peaks during this phase, enhancing motivation and the brain's reward system and making it easier to engage in productive habits, stay motivated, and align actions with goals. Estrogen also influences emotional resonance and empathy through mirror neurons.[6] During estrogen-dominant phases, we may experience heightened sensitivity to our environment and relationships, deepening inspiration and connection. This emotional engagement helps align thoughts, feelings, and behaviors with personal desires and aspirations, amplifying the effectiveness of our creative endeavors and manifestation practices.

Awaken Phase Practices

What follows is a collection of optional activities for you to incorporate into your Awaken phases going forward. As you become more and more familiar with the energy of this phase, you might like to add your own ideas and exercises to this selection. Like your own personal manifestation catalog, you can choose which practices resonate with you. Delve into them during your follicular phase (pre-ovulation) toward the end of your menstruation if you're following your menstrual cycle, or around the time of the waxing crescent moon if you're following the moon cycle. This is when the natural universal energies best support planning and initiating. You might also like to try some these during the season of Spring, or really at any time the mood strikes. You might want to keep things simple and try just one of these practices each time you arrive at your Awaken phase (about once a month). It's up to you!

Cycle Habits Optimized (Stacking, Combining, and Enhancing)

What could be better than getting into alignment with soul-nourishing habits? Your skin is glowing, your bank account is growing, your body feels strong, your heart is full, and your mind is at ease. As good as this feels, though, know that it can get even better! What if engaging with your habits becomes fun? This collection of three exercises will have you mastering the art of Cycle Habits and supercharging your results as you optimize your time, biohack your way to wellness, and enjoy the journey.

Developing habits can be challenging. As we explored in the previous chapter, our brains tend to be wired to repeat behaviors and ways of thinking that are already familiar to us, so starting any new habit will require more focus and attention upfront, and then thanks to neuroplasticity we can learn to adapt to new behaviors and return to them with greater ease once they become familiar. But before we dig any further into neuroscience, let me tell you about Katya.

On a rainy London evening, I was sitting at a small table waiting for friends at a private members' club when Katya walked in. From her cascading long blond hair down to her high-heeled Louboutins, her presence drew everyone's attention. She shimmied out of a fur-trimmed Dolce & Gabbana full-length coat and walked toward me. I'd been guarding the four-seat table for 30 minutes as I waited for my friends to arrive, but as Katya slunk into the seat across from me, I simply smiled. "Hi, darling, I'm Katya." We talked briefly about fashion but were quickly interrupted by two well-dressed businessmen.

"Good evening, ladies, may we order you a drink?" I smiled and told them I'd love a cosmopolitan. "No, darling, you want *champagne*," Katya interrupted. A moment later a waiter appeared with two frosty glasses of bubbly. One of the men gestured to the seat next to Katya and asked if he could sit down, but Katya's handbag was on the seat. With a swipe of her blond locks and a pout she stated, "It's Chanel, darling, I can't put it on the floor."

Like Katya, if the human brain had a theme song it would be "It's expensive to be me." In metabolic terms, the brain is our most expensive organ. It consumes roughly 20 percent of the body's energy at rest, yet accounts for only about 2 percent of total body weight, using approximately 320 calories per day to sustain its constant activity.[7]

The techniques that follow will help you integrate new habits with existing ones so you can reserve your mental energy for tasks that require absolute focus. That way, you can leverage the strong synaptic connections and neural networks that you already possess. Get ready to amplify your impact! Set aside at least 15 minutes for each of the three exercises. Feel free to do them all together, or at separate times. They do not have to be done in sequence.

Cycle Habit Stacking

Coming into alignment with healthy habits can boost our confidence and wellness. If you've been enjoying your habits and returning to them consistently (though not necessarily every day), then you're probably feeling good. Really good. And we know that when something's good—like a matcha pancake, a gold bracelet, a hundred-dollar bill, or an issue of *Vogue*—it's only natural to want to stack it up and enjoy the multiplication of goodness. Grab your journal and follow the steps below to begin habit stacking.

1. Choose a habit, action, or routine you are already doing or one you want to do that will be easy for you (perhaps something you've already had success with in the past).

2. On a fresh page in your journal, write what your habit is exactly halfway down the page, with equal space above it and below it.

3. What other beneficial actions could you do before you perform this habit? Write your ideas on the top half of the page, above the habit.

4. What other beneficial actions could you do after you complete this habit? Write your ideas on the bottom half of the page, below your habit.

5. Circle the ideas on either side of your existing habit that you want to try "stacking."

6. Schedule performing this new, stacked habit for a time when it makes the most sense to test it out. It will feel uncomfortable at first and you may forget the sequence, but keep persisting and perfecting it so you can add it to your Cycle Habits.

Example:
Ideas to do before: Apply a hair oil treatment, do body brushing, give yourself a facial, trim the ends of your hair during the waxing moon, use a scalp brush when shampooing, perform a gua sha facial before your shower, take a sauna or red-light therapy session, do a sweaty workout
Habit: Wash hair in the shower
Ideas to do after: Do self-massage, apply body lotion, exfoliate your body while conditioning your hair, do a cold-water rinse of your hair, blast cold and then warm water on yourself in the shower, apply a hair treatment, change your pillowcase, apply self-tanning lotion, do a manicure or pedicure

Cycle Habit Combining

Habit combining is all about augmenting and enriching the habits you are already doing so you are achieving multiple goals at the same time. You'll need your journal and at least 15 minutes to explore this exercise. Follow the steps below.

1. At the top of a fresh page in your journal, write down one habit related to the body. This could be some type of movement, exercise, self-care, or relaxation.

2. Review the questions below and add any ideas you might have to your journal.

   Can I use light weights or resistance bands while I do this workout?

   Can I add warmth or heat to this practice?

   Can I do this outdoors, near an open window, or in the sun?

   Can I wear special clothing or bands to encourage sweating?

   Can I do this in bare feet on soil, water, or sand?

   Can I listen to a motivational show or podcast while doing this?

   Can I wear a fitness tracker, heart-rate monitor, or step counter?

   Can I add anything to my head or face, such as a facial mask or headphones?

   Can I lie on something that stimulates my body, like an acupressure or a PEMF mat?

   Can I use a blanket or weighted blanket to support relaxation?

What other healthy actions or habits can I do while this is happening?

Can I add music or binaural beats for relaxation?

How can I make this a holistic wellness practice?

Can I add anything to a chair or where I sit?

Can I do deep breathing during this activity?

Can I stimulate my muscles in some way?

What else can I add to this habit to optimize it?

3. After you've written down all your ideas, create combinations of several different actions together and try them out as part of your Cycle Habits.

4. Repeat this exercise for any additional habits you want to explore.

Example:

Establish an at-home spa day once a week where you combine treatments that take time to "marinate." For example, in the morning, apply self-tanning lotion as well as a hair mask and a facial mask and paint your toenails. Several hours later you will have achieved a lot, all in the same time period.

There are endless ways to combine habits. Make a list of all the habits you'd do if you had all the free time in the world, then try blending some of them together. Have fun with this!

Cycle Habit Enhancing

Don't you just love immersive experiences? Watching a movie in IMAX, journeying through a ride at a theme park, or running through a superbloom field in Spring? Or how about giving something a five-star level of attention to detail? Finding a mini fridge at the gym with a stack of refreshing eucalyptus-scented face towels, or an elegant glass dispenser filled with lemon, cucumber, and mint spa water? Well, I can't promise you we'll go to *that* level of awesomeness (unless you're Katya from London), but you'll be using all your five senses to enhance your Cycle Habits, because the best, most effective habits are the ones that are kept in rotation over the long term—or even for life! So you will definitely want to make them as enjoyable and uplifting for your mind, body, and soul as possible.

When I had trouble keeping up with my skincare routine, I tried moving it to different times of the day, but I was still getting bored by having to spend 10 to 15 minutes in front of the mirror as I did my gua sha facial and applied my serums and lotions. I really wanted to enjoy the benefits of this, but I was struggling to be consistent. I ended up adding a small acrylic shelf right under my makeup mirror so I could put my iPad there and watch YouTube videos while I was doing my skincare routine. This has worked out great, because I no longer have the dreaded FOMO while being tucked away in the bathroom staring at the mirror and doing repetitive upward strokes on my face. I also added an essential oil diffuser with mood lighting for a spalike vibe. Bliss!

Grab your journal and reserve about 15 minutes for this exercise. Follow the steps to begin.

1. On a fresh page in your journal, write down a habit you'd like to enhance to make it more enjoyable.
2. Review the questions below and add any ideas you might have to your journal.
   What will I want to watch while I am doing this habit?
   What will I want to smell as I am doing this habit?
   How could I entertain my taste buds as I am doing this habit?

Who can I invite to join me while I do this habit?

How can I make this habit more comfortable?

How can I make this habit more fun?

What will I want to feel on my skin while I do this habit?

How can I make this a more stimulating experience?

How can I make this a more relaxing experience?

What can I do to enhance the environment where this habit takes place?

What would give me good vibes as I do this habit?

How can I make this a more soulful experience?

How can I bring more love into this experience?

How can I bring more fun, happiness, and joy into this experience?

How can I bring more self-care into this experience?

What time of day feels best for doing this habit?

Could this be part of a longer ritual or routine?

What can I drink or add to my water to drink while I do this?

Can I make this a low-stress activity?

3. After you've written down all your ideas, select the perfect enhancements for your habit and try them out as part of your Cycle Habits.

4. Repeat this exercise for any additional habits you want to explore.

Example:

Cycle Habit: Meditation

Enhancement ideas: Designate a small area as the place where you'll meditate regularly. Use a decorative footstool, chair, or floor cushion that might be stashed away when not in use. Add a small table or shelf to hold spiritual books, crystals, essential oils, or other meditation tools. Listen to soothing music or guided meditations through headphones to help yourself focus and relax. Add an inspirational element such as mood lighting, a small fountain, a salt crystal lamp, artwork, or a vase with flowers. Burn palo santo before beginning. Follow it with a tea ritual.

Supportive Structures

Our foray into stacking, combining, and enhancing our Cycle Habits was all about *fun*, and now, as we explore Supportive Structures for our habits, it becomes all about *ease*. Yes, even the healthiest habits get to be fun and easy. Investing time and attention in the creation of Supportive Structures up front will make your new habits easier to accomplish and stick with over the long term, which will help you build momentum. Supportive Structures also relieve you of the burden of having to expend so much energy on sheer willpower alone. Your Supportive Structures can serve you for years to come so your habits run seamlessly and you enjoy the compounding effects and leveled-up results of living a life you love.

I have a confession to make. My current lifestyle revolves, quite literally, around my Cycle Habits. Over the years and the cycles, I've continued to invest in my Supportive Structures, and it has kept me living a life of wellness and fun. Thanks to Supportive Structures like a well-organized, dedicated space for my workout clothing and accessories, I'm ready to hit the hiking trails, beach, or fitness class at a moment's notice. There are certain activities I keep up with almost daily, and there are other habits I do in rotation within my cycle. I am able to remain open, curious, and flexible about new ideas and ways of doing things and at the same time enjoy the core mind, body, and soul habits that I *know* work well for me now and will serve me in years to come so I can be healthy, happy, and abundant. As I mastered my habits, people started to ask me what kinds of wellness practices I was doing and how I managed to achieve certain things, as well as comment on my energy levels. It's not about the specific wellness practices, or the workouts, diet, or mindset tools. My secret is the Cycle Habit Supportive Structures that I have put in place and enhanced over time. They keep me inspired, consistent, and able to do the things I love with ease. But that wasn't always the case!

In my earlier days of attempting to create habits, a practice would enter my life for a short while only to exit soon after. My life was like a revolving door of habits. Nothing really stuck. I had a broad idea of the types of habits I wanted to follow, but my resolve wasn't strong, so it didn't take much to derail me. If I missed a day of doing a certain habit, I tended to give up on it and feel like a failure. When I look back at how I used to spend my time before I had my Cycle Habits and Supportive Structures in place, it seems like a child was in charge.

On weekends you could find me pursuing any number of random energy-exerting activities, often centered around buying things I didn't need. On one particular Sunday afternoon I found myself aimlessly wandering the aisles of a huge arts-and-crafts store, armed with a 20 percent discount coupon and looking for trouble. I turned the corner into an aisle I'd never ventured down before and that's when I became absolutely mesmerized. Perhaps it's the Virgo energy in my chart, but I absolutely love to organize things and collect items in various colors. There before me was an entire wall stocked with what must have been thousands of neatly packaged little strands of beads. Some were precious stones like rose quartz or turquoise, some were sparkly, some were polished, some were faceted, and others had a natural pebble shape with marbling. From cream to pale yellow to orange, pink, crimson, purple, blue, and beyond, the entire wall was color coordinated. I felt like Dorothy having just arrived in the Land of Oz. I struggled to focus my eyes, because I truly did not know where to look. Or where to start. But I knew I had to have them. I grabbed my basket and started filling it with packet after packet of colorful beads. When I got home and surveyed my bounty, I stared at them and wondered what I was going to use them for. That's right, I had purchased a basketful of beads with zero plan in mind for what to do with them. I reasoned that I could make bracelets for friends' birthdays, and to match some of my outfits, and maybe even sell some online. Three days later after receiving an e-mail from the store with a $40 coupon based on my recent splurge, I doubled down and went back to purchase jewelry-making tools and four extra-large acrylic bead storage containers to display them aesthetically. I assigned color themes for the containers and poured each individual bead packet into its section. When I was done I admired my bead collection with satisfaction (and guilt). When I selected a few beads of various hues, materials, and shapes to combine into a bracelet, I felt like Kelly Wearstler in her studio preparing a design palette to show a client.

It's been several years since then and I have probably made seven bracelets in total. While there's nothing wrong with splurging on creative pursuits and following your joy, in this instance, I was not acting in alignment with how I truly wanted to be using my time, energy, or money to bring value to my life or the lives of others. Instead, I got carried away by the pretty colors and shapes and then filed them away in boxes, quite literally.

These days, I make sure to indulge my playful side (and my love of color) regularly with things that truly feed my soul and feminine essence, like swimming in the ocean under a vivid sunset; painting my nails; creating vibrant smoothie bowls and crudité platters; helping friends with interior-design projects; painting an artwork on canvas for my office; creating YouTube videos; baking and decorating cakes for friends and family; creating websites, ebooks, and digital templates; and collecting color-coordinated workout gear (clothing, shoes, caps, mini backpacks), things I actually *use regularly* to up-level my health and wellness. I now enjoy having some structure around my creativity and use it to bring value to my life.

Can you see the tweak I made here? Instead of creating energy leaks by aimlessly indulging my whims and letting myself be pulled in the direction of whatever shiny object catches my attention, I now have deeply aligned mind, body, and soul habits and Supportive Structures that I pour my creativity into. This is what creates a compounding effect in my life, expanding my fulfillment, health, abundance, love, and happiness. I'm investing my precious life-force energy in myself, my loved ones, and the work I share with others.

Creating your Cycle Habits and Supportive Structures is something that can unfold over time. Have fun experimenting with the types of habits you want to adopt, and the various ways in which you can support them to make your life flow with ease while feeling fun and inspiring at the same time. Follow the steps to get started:

1. Begin by choosing three habits you'd like to try as part of your Cycle Habits system.
2. Taking one habit at a time, imagine all the things you would need to have in place to be able to make this

habit flow and reduce any resistance to starting it. Run through performing the habit in your mind from start to finish. What has to happen before, during, and after you do it? What needs to happen first? Think about all the steps that come after that. What can you do after doing it to make it easy to do again the next time?

3. Write down all your ideas, including things you might need to invest in at a future time to make your habits easy to start and easy to maintain. You might want to make a plan to put away a small amount of money each month to invest in your Supportive Structures over time. Here are some examples:

Example 1:
Cycle Habit: Make a superfood smoothie
Supportive Structure: Set up a space in the pantry and use labeled containers to store any powdered ingredients so they are easy to access. Subscribe for automatic monthly delivery of certain ingredients. Purchase containers such as sugar dispensers for any powdered ingredients that need to be refrigerated so it's quick and easy to pour them into the blender. Dedicate space in the fridge and freezer for produce containers for the fresh and frozen ingredients. Download a grocery app to keep track of when you need to buy more fresh ingredients.

Example 2:
Cycle Habit: Perform body brushing
Supportive Structure: Set up a dedicated area near the shower for a body brush and body oils, lotions, and self-massage tools to use before or after showering. This could be a small, decorative garden stool or a shelf to hang brushes under with oils and lotions placed on top.

Example 3:

Cycle Habit: Work out at home
Supportive Structure: Research and select online classes to try. Create a small corner or cabinet near your exercise space to store equipment such as a yoga mat, resistance bands, light weights, or a Pilates ball. Schedule uninterrupted time and put devices on silent mode during the sessions. Have a small towel ready for use during sweaty workouts. Use a mini foam roller or self-massage tools after workouts. Play upbeat music, or diffuse uplifting essential oils while working out. Have a dedicated water bottle to use when working out. Change into comfortable workout clothing in preparation for working out.

Biohack Your Habits by Aligning with Circadian Rhythms

Although as women we beat to more of a monthly drum, we're also governed by daily circadian rhythms, so we'll typically experience a natural energy boost powered by the cortisol awakening response in the morning that tapers off in the afternoon and evening as melatonin production rises.[8] With this in mind, you might consider "doing the difficult thing" in the morning. If maintaining an energy-intensive habit like exercise is a priority but feels difficult to sustain, try scheduling it during your natural energy peaks—early in the day during the Awaken and Thrive phases of your cycle. This is the first of many tips that we can glean from the world of biohacking.

During my studies at the Institute for Integrative Nutrition, visiting faculty member and biohacking expert Ben Greenfield described biohacking as "the practice of using any tool or strategy to get the body and brain to operate more efficiently." Biohacking uses science, technology, and lifestyle changes to optimize physical and mental performance, health, and well-being. It often involves experimenting with nutrition, exercise, sleep, and other habits to "hack" the body's biology for better outcomes. While biohacking embraces modern technology like red-light therapy and wearable devices, it also draws inspiration from ancestral rituals like fasting, cold exposure, and practices aligned with nature's rhythms.

Biohacking with circadian rhythms involves aligning your lifestyle with the body's natural 24-hour cycles to optimize your wellness and energy. The circadian rhythm regulates vital functions such as sleep, metabolism, and hormone production. By aligning activities with this biological clock, you can reduce stress, stabilize mood, improve focus and productivity, boost immune function and metabolism, promote hormone balance, and enhance overall vitality.

As we explored in Chapter 1, our bodies are learning to adapt to a time of evolutionary mismatch, and it's easy to feel misaligned in our natural energy cycles and disconnected from nature. Disruptions to circadian rhythms can significantly impact our health due to the intricate connection between the body's internal clock and hormonal systems. Irregular sleep schedules, high levels of stress, and exposure to artificial light during evening hours can all desynchronize the circadian rhythm. This misalignment interferes with the regular secretion of hormones such as melatonin. As women, we may experience amplified effects from these disruptions due to our shifting hormones throughout the menstrual cycle. Over time, chronic circadian misalignment may lead to issues such as mood swings, heightened anxiety, and irritability, as well as physical health challenges like insulin resistance, weight gain, and increased risk of cardiovascular or metabolic disorders. These effects can be particularly pronounced during hormonal transitions like pregnancy and perimenopause. It's important that we reduce our exposure to the long-term health risks associated with circadian misalignment. This is where biohacking can help us to not only cope better with today's stressors, but also make simple shifts to realign with natural energies in order to thrive.

So, what can we learn from seasoned biohackers about leveraging the natural circadian rhythm to our advantage? Here are some tips to help you biohack your habits.

- Morning sunlight exposure stimulates the release of cortisol and serotonin, hormones that promote wakefulness and improve mood. Upon waking, open your blinds or curtains to let in natural sunlight, helping to align and regulate your circadian rhythm.

- With the natural rise of energy early in the day, you may want to make your morning routine the time when you do all the things that will set you up to have a successful day instead of trying to get them done the night before. It can be difficult to get through a complicated routine in the evening, when your body is naturally preparing to relax.

- Consider incorporating short bursts of cold-water exposure in the morning to stimulate circulation and boost alertness. While cold exposure can be energizing, extended exposure may not be ideal for women, as it can stress the body and overtax the adrenal glands. Instead, opt for shorter bursts, like splashing your face with cold water, using an ice roller on your face and body, or alternating quick bursts of warm and cold water in the shower. Since most research on cold plunging is based on men (whose hormonal landscape is vastly different from women's), it's important to listen to your body and keep the practice gentle to support your hormonal and adrenal health.

- Eating meals during daylight hours aligns digestion with metabolic rhythms. Avoid late-night eating to prevent disruptions in insulin sensitivity and other metabolic processes. Choose local, pesticide-free seasonal produce whenever possible and avoid processed foods.

- If you practice fasting, consider aligning it with your hormonal cycle by opting for shorter fasting windows during the luteal phase (when your body may need more nourishment) and experimenting with longer windows during the follicular phase, when energy levels and metabolic flexibility are typically higher. If you're dealing with adrenal fatigue, consider skipping fasts altogether and exploring plant-based cleanses instead. For those who choose to fast, approach it with care—start gradually and allow your body ample time to adjust.

- Being in touch with the natural rhythms, ecosystems, and energies of nature can help us build our immunity through habits like earthing and spending time in nature. Spending time outdoors not only connects us to the Earth's natural energies but also helps to reset and synchronize our body's internal clock, boosting resilience and vitality. (See page 99 for more about earthing.)

- Avoid delaying Cycle Habits until later in the day or overloading your evenings with tasks when your energy is naturally waning, as this can make it harder to follow through. Instead, save high-energy habits for earlier in the day and focus on more restful, calming activities in the evening to align with your body's natural rhythm.

- Going to bed and waking up at the same times daily helps stabilize circadian rhythms. This predictability strengthens the sleep-wake cycle, improving both the quality and duration of sleep. A good night's sleep is essential for overall health, immune activity, and longevity, affecting everything from cognitive function to stress level and long-term well-being.

- In the evenings, create a digital sunset by setting your devices to filter out blue light, or use blue-light-filtering eyeglasses after sunset. If you have a voice-activated device or smart home hub, you could also adjust the setting on your smart lights to dim automatically after sunset. This will help your body naturally wind down and prepare for restorative sleep by encouraging melatonin production. Red LED clip-on reading lamps can also feel soothing for late-night reading before bed. Allow for longer sleep periods during the darker Winter months.

- Plan relaxing habits as part of your evening routine to promote better sleep quality. Practices like reading, journaling, meditating, deep breathing, self-massage with body oils, or gentle stretching can help you wind down before bed, easing tension and improving sleep quality.

- Try heat therapies in the evening to relax and recover after a busy day. Spend time in a sauna or a sauna blanket to sweat out toxins or use infrared light panels, heated massage tools, or heating pads to help soothe sore muscles. Warm showers and baths can help to relax muscles prior to going to sleep.

- Create a conducive sleep environment by making your bedroom like a cave—dark, cool, and quiet. Keeping the bedroom cool signals the body to wind down for sleep because lower temperatures naturally promote the release of melatonin. You can also eliminate distractions such as electronic devices and excessive noise to further enhance your body's ability to relax and sync with its circadian rhythm for a restful night.

Cultivating awareness of the natural energies around you will help you time your actions and habits to best suit your body's needs, supporting optimal energy and rest.

Exercise:

Grab your journal and follow the steps to align your habits with your circadian rhythms:

1. What important habits or routines would you like to get done in the mornings to leverage your peak natural energy?

2. How can you make the best use of evening habits when your natural energy is waning?

3. What other ways can you think of to align with your circadian rhythm?

Stimulants and Energy Balance

Many caffeine drinkers start their day with coffee, green tea, or a chai tea latte immediately upon waking. However, this coincides with the body's natural cortisol peak, typically 30 to 45 minutes after waking, when energy is already high. If you're looking to reduce caffeine reliance, consider delaying consumption until later in the morning or at midday, when the cortisol level naturally dips. Drinking caffeine with or shortly after eating food can also help to buffer the effects. Chocolate, a sneaky source of caffeine, can impact sleep if consumed late in the day or evening. Indulging in that square of dark chocolate late at night might be undermining your attempts at a restful night's sleep. As if that wasn't enough bad news, an evening glass of red wine could also be a culprit when it comes to sleep issues. Alcohol can act as a double agent, calming the nervous system at first, but then causing a stimulating effect that can interfere with deep and REM sleep.[9] If you're sensitive to caffeine or struggle with sleep, opt for noncaffeinated treats in the evening, such as a carob bar, medjool dates filled with nut butter, a baked apple, an herbal tea latte, or banana "nice cream." Instead of alcohol, try a magnesium-infused cherry mocktail, a glass of nonalcoholic wine, or another functional beverage suited for rest and relaxation.

Living in Alignment

When your habits reflect your core values, you create a sense of harmony and fulfillment in your life. This alignment fortifies your actions and builds confidence over time as you channel the energies available to you toward your dreams and aspirations. Your values help to shape the foundation for your "why"—the deeper motivations driving your manifestation journey. By anchoring your behaviors to these guiding principles, you'll feel better equipped to overcome doubts that may arise when progress feels stagnant or elusive.

Do your day-to-day actions reflect your values and align with the life you want to live? Your values shape your decisions, your priorities, and the energy you bring to different areas of your life. This exercise is designed to help you identify outdated values, embrace new ones, and align your daily actions with who you're becoming.

Exercise:

1. In your journal, create a table with three columns, or use the table below.

2. List your desires in the first column. For each desire, write the related values that have driven your actions in the past in the second column. In the third column write the values that align with the outcome you wish to manifest now.

DESIRE	PAST VALUE	PRESENT VALUE
Create a business	Security, avoiding risk	Creativity, sharing my gifts
Attract/improve a relationship	Independence, being in control	Vulnerability, empathy

3. In your journal, create statements to reinforce each value that you wish to upgrade:

- Where once I valued _____ [e.g., working late hours], I now value _____ [e.g., work-life balance].

- Where once I valued _____ [e.g., burning calories], I now value _____ [e.g., building strength, mobility, and longevity].

4. Which of your new, upgraded values feels the *most* inspiring and energizing to you right now? _____
_____

5. Think of a habit that aligns with your new, upgraded value and add it to your Cycle Habits Tracker.

> Reminder: *Consistently* doesn't have to equal *daily*. When adding a habit to your Cycle Habits Tracker, you're tracking it only on days when it aligns with your body's energy. This approach allows you to focus on what feels right rather than on striving to "check it off the list" each day.

Longevity Habits in Rotation

Engaging in natural, enjoyable habits today can plant the seeds for long-term wellness and fill you with optimism for what's to come. Here, I've combined insights from Blue Zone studies of regions where people live the longest with evidence-based lifestyle medicine approaches I learned at Harvard Medical School to come up with a powerful set of recommendations for well-being and longevity. Viewing wellness holistically—beyond what's on our plate—reveals that true nourishment encompasses how we feed our minds and souls, not just our bodies.

Eat the Rainbow

A colorful, plant-predominant diet filled with whole, nutrient-packed foods like fruits, vegetables, whole grains, legumes, and nuts is a great way to support long-term health and well-being. These foods are rich in antioxidants, fiber, and colorful phytonutrients that help reduce inflammation, support a healthy gut, and protect against chronic diseases. Prioritizing homemade meals and cutting back on processed foods, sugary drinks, and sodium mirror the natural, unprocessed diets enjoyed by communities who live longer, healthier lives.

Move Your Body

Incorporate regular, moderate movement in ways that feel natural and enjoyable, such as walking, gardening, or dancing. Focus on consistent activity that integrates seamlessly into your routines rather than relying solely on structured workouts. Movement throughout the day—like walking after meals, taking the stairs, stretching, and engaging in household tasks—can support cardiovascular health, build muscle, and boost mental well-being, making physical activity both sustainable and beneficial.

Connect with Others

Cultivating strong relationships and social networks is key for health and longevity. Research from Harvard shows that close family ties and community connections can reduce stress and enhance mental health, contributing to a longer, more fulfilling life.[10] Social support is important for overall well-being, helping to build mental resilience and aiding in physical recovery. To nurture these connections, make quality time with loved ones a priority through activities like family meals, gatherings with friends, and community events. Regularly set aside time to deepen these relationships and maintain strong social networks with like-minded people.

Stress-Reduction Practices

Practice mindfulness and stress-reduction techniques to manage stress and promote mental clarity. In many cultures with long lifespans, daily rituals like prayer, meditation, and relaxation practices are key for reducing stress, fostering calm, and enhancing well-being. Incorporating mindfulness—through meditation, journaling, or other practices—helps reduce blood pressure, regulate your stress response, and bring peace to your day.[11]

Purpose and Passion

Finding and maintaining a sense of purpose in life—through meaningful work, hobbies, or volunteer activities—can greatly impact longevity and health. Studies from Harvard and Blue Zones show that having a clear sense of purpose is associated with longer life expectancy and better health outcomes.[12] Cultivating a sense of purpose, often referred to as *ikigai* in Japanese, can improve mental health, reduce stress, and enhance overall well-being. Reflecting on what brings you joy and meaning and setting small, aligned goals can help you reconnect with your purpose daily.

Follow Your Curiosity

Engaging in activities that challenge the brain—such as doing puzzles, reading, learning new skills, and following your curiosity on a variety of topics—can protect against cognitive decline and contribute to increased longevity. These activities stimulate neuroplasticity, helping the brain maintain connections and adapt to changes over time. Being a lifelong learner supports mental sharpness and adaptability, reducing the risk of neurodegenerative diseases and enhancing overall brain health.[13] Regular mental stimulation combined with curiosity about diverse interests can help to foster a longer, healthier life.

Exercise:
Think of one habit that you believe will set you up for long-term wellness and add it to your Cycle Habits Tracker to begin incorporating it in rotation during your cycles.

Breaking Through Resistance

Midway between the new moon and the full moon, the first quarter moon emerges in the sky, her face half illuminated by light and half in shadow. Don't let her cutesy black-and-white-cookie appearance fool you; the quarter moon's stark contrast between dark and light reveals a deeper truth to her nature and value in our lives. Her duality reminds us that for all our high-spirited determination and positivity in working toward our goals, there will inevitably be times when fears, doubts, and uncertainties lurk. At these times, we may perceive not just the excitement and anticipation of the things we wish to manifest, but also the effort it's going to take to achieve them. Just as the quarter moon's illumination shines a light on hidden parts, we may cast questions about our dedication, commitment, or motivation on ourselves. She's here to aid us in transforming dark into light. That's her secret.

If you're following your menstrual cycle, then the elevation of estrogen during this follicular phase will foster confidence and assertiveness in the face of any friction. You may feel more open to trying new things and exploring new opportunities.

Whether you're aligning with the moon or your menstrual cycle, the Awaken phase is an ideal time to strengthen your resolve, take calculated risks, and break through challenges, because the energy that's available to you supports outward engagement, curiosity, and tenacity. Any resistance you encounter during this phase isn't meant to halt your progress but rather to help you build clarity and strengthen your commitment to growth despite obstacles. When it comes to following through on your Cycle Habits, the energy of this phase invites the building of resilience and the willingness to push through initial discomfort or hesitation. This is an opportunity to course correct as you gain insights about what does and doesn't work. In this exercise you'll examine where you've encountered resistance in forming new habits. Are there specific behaviors, thoughts, or external factors that have made it difficult? By identifying these, you can address the root cause and find ways to adjust rather than abandon your habit. This is also a good time to evaluate whether you're putting unnecessary pressure on yourself to be perfect, which can create internal resistance. Friction of any kind can be a sign that small tweaks are needed. For instance, if a daily meditation habit is hard to sustain, perhaps the timing or setting needs adjusting.

Exercise:

Turn to a fresh page in your journal and choose three or more of these journal prompts to help yourself break through resistance:

- What challenges am I anticipating as I begin or continue my Cycle Habits?

- In what ways could I introduce accountability as I pursue my goals? Would it help to enlist a friend or another person in the process?

- What distractions might arise, and how will I deal with them?

- What excites me the most about the manifestations of my desires?
- What have I learned so far during the Awaken phase, and what still needs to be done?
- Where might I be off track, and what's the next small step I can take to realign?
- When I have overcome significant obstacles in the past, what strategies did I use, and how can I apply them to my current challenge?
- How can I cultivate more patience and resilience when facing setbacks or challenges?
- What does success look like to me, and how can I stay focused on that vision even when I encounter obstacles?
- Are there any new practices, habits, or routines that I could implement to help myself maintain a positive mindset and overcome challenges?

By exploring these questions during the Awaken phase, you can make yourself more resilient, adaptable, and aligned with your intentions in practicing your habits, setting a strong foundation as you move forward.

Small, consistent actions can have a compounding effect over time. Acknowledge your progress, and celebrate small victories. This can reinforce your motivation and help you sustain your Cycle Habits beyond any initial resistance.

Cycle Habits for Hormonal Harmony

Feeling a little hormonally off-balance? There's a lot we can do with lifestyle changes to enhance our body's natural ability to maintain a healthy hormone balance. When our hormones are dysregulated, meaning out of balance, we can experience symptoms like irregular periods, mood swings, fatigue, night sweats, weight fluctuation, trouble sleeping, brain fog, low libido, hair loss, and more. By tuning in to your body's natural rhythms and creating balance with nourishing practices and lifestyle habits, you can pave the way for greater hormonal harmony.

Today, it's quite common to experience irregular periods or challenges with thyroid health. Up to 35 percent of women experience some type of menstrual cycle irregularity.[15] The American Thyroid Association estimates that one in eight women will develop a thyroid disorder during their lifetime, and women are five to eight times more likely than men to have thyroid problems.[16] The thyroid is a small, butterfly-shaped gland located at the front of the neck that plays a powerful role in regulating metabolism, energy level, and hormonal balance throughout the body. So how can we show her some love? By embracing a holistic approach to self-care, you're helping to safeguard this queenly gland that plays a vital role in regulating your hormones. Your thyroid isn't asking you to race, push, overdo, or overextend yourself. Instead, she wants you to find balance and flow and to care for yourself in the most loving, sustainable way. Here are some holistic lifestyle approaches for supporting hormone balance and healthy thyroid function.

Gut Health

A healthy gut is essential for metabolizing hormones, particularly estrogen. The gut-brain axis and the hypothalamic-pituitary-adrenal axis are key systems linking gut health and hormonal balance, especially in women. When your gut microbes are out of balance, it can affect your menstrual cycle, fertility, mood, weight, and more. A healthy gut also helps regulate insulin production and blood sugar level. To support gut health and hormonal balance, try reducing gluten and processed, sugary, and fried foods. Focus on a fiber-rich diet highlighting organic produce like cruciferous vegetables, leafy greens, and fruits. Include hormone-free meats, whole grains, legumes, and fermented foods or probiotics. Brazil nuts provide selenium, and sea vegetables and wild-caught fish provide iodine and omega-3 fatty acids, all of which are helpful for thyroid health.

Reduce Stress

Chronic stress can interfere with thyroid function, depleting essential resources like magnesium and selenium. An elevated cortisol level caused by ongoing stress disrupts estrogen and progesterone production, which can result in irregular periods, PMS, and other hormone imbalances. High cortisol can also slow thyroid hormone production, potentially contributing to hypothyroidism. Relaxation practices such as deep breathing, yin yoga, meditation, journaling, and spending quality time with friends can be effective ways to manage stress. Grounding activities like walking barefoot on the earth and enjoying Epsom salts baths are also beneficial. When it comes to exercise, engage in physical activities that don't spike cortisol, such as resistance training, Pilates, yoga, or walking. Mindful eating, breath work, meditation, and gentle exercise support adrenal health and help keep stress in check.

Detoxify

Detoxification plays a key role in thyroid health because toxins, especially heavy metals, can block iodine uptake and disrupt hormone conversion. Support detoxification by adhering to a clean diet, drinking filtered water, and minimizing radiation and electromagnetic field (EMF) exposure. Reduce EMFs by turning off your Wi-Fi at night and using EMF blockers. Reducing your use of chemicals and plastics protects the thyroid and endocrine system from toxic disruptors like PCBs, perchlorate, dioxins, triclosan, BPA, and phthalates. Common sources of these chemicals include household products like shampoos, laundry detergents, plastic food wraps and containers, and even furniture. Opt for nontoxic cleaning products, use glass instead of plastic for food and beverages, and purchase sustainably sourced foods. Make mindful choices to reduce products like antibacterial soaps and flame-retardant furniture. Supporting your thyroid with proper nutrition like natural sources of iodine as well as stress management can help mitigate the effects of environmental toxins.

Minimize Radiation

Radiation can impact thyroid function by mimicking hormones or disrupting iodine uptake, potentially slowing thyroid activity and affecting hormonal balance. To reduce exposure, limit use of devices that emit radiation and speak to your health care practitioner about avoiding unnecessary X-ray procedures. Keep phones away from your body, use earbuds for calls, and switch to airplane mode when possible. Choose a pat-down instead of going through airport X-ray scanners.

Prioritize Sleep

Establish a consistent bedtime routine and create a digital sunset in your home. Reduce artificial light at night, especially blue light from screens, which can interfere with your circadian clock. You can also set your devices to filter out blue light or transition to night mode after sunset to promote restful sleep and hormonal balance. Spending time outdoors in natural sunlight for a few minutes, especially in the early morning, can also synchronize you with your circadian rhythms.

Practice Lunaception

Try this holistic practice that has been used to support hormonal balance: On the night before, the night of, and the night after the full moon, allow natural moonlight into your bedroom by opening your curtains or blinds. If that's not possible, sleep with a nightlight or soft light turned on during those three nights. This practice, known as Lunaception, may help regulate the menstrual cycle. You might also enjoy moon bathing by sitting or standing in the moonlight for 10 to 15 minutes on these nights, possibly combining it with meditation or visualization of your desired manifestations coming to fruition.

Avoid Risky Substances

Support your overall wellness with lifestyle medicine, which emphasizes avoiding substances that can harm hormone, liver, and gut health. Reducing or eliminating alcohol, refined sugars, processed foods, conventional meats, smoking, and drugs can lower your risk of disease and help to nourish your body's natural systems for lasting health.

Supplements and Testing

Consider incorporating supplements into your routine, but consult with a health care practitioner first to ensure that there are no contraindications to taking them along with your current medications or vitamins. Choose reputable brands without unnecessary additives and GMOs, and conduct third-party testing for toxins and heavy metals since supplements are not regulated by the FDA. If you suspect you have a hormone imbalance or thyroid dysfunction, ask your health care practitioner for lab tests, such as a DUTCH hormone test, or for a screening for blood count, liver function, blood sugar, cholesterol, and vitamin levels—all of which can impact hormone health.

Exercise:

Reflect on the ways in which your current Cycle Habits may serve your hormonal health and overall well-being. Are there any new habits you wish to add or actions you'd like to take to further support your hormonal harmony and wellness?

Lifestyle Awakening

Enjoy experimenting with these lifestyle-enhancing ideas during the Awaken phase.

Mind

- Diffuse essential oils with energizing and uplifting qualities, such as rosemary, grapefruit, orange, and peppermint.

- Socialize, connect with friends, and spend time with like-minded people in mastermind sessions, classes, and groups to share ideas and collaborate on solutions and actions to excel in business and other areas.

- Focus on communication, publishing, or social media projects at this time to align with uplifting energies.

Body

- Consider doing a short detox during this phase, especially if you are aligning with your menstrual cycle because the follicular phase is a time when we naturally have less of an appetite compared with later in the cycle.

- Embrace athletic wear. Be ready to move your body and flow with the uplifting energies in this phase, whether it's by doing some muscle toning or a sweaty workout to expel toxins.

- Indulge yourself in a sauna session, body scrub, or exfoliation to aid detoxification.

- Consider meals that incorporate seeds, high-fiber cruciferous veggies, healthy fats, and fermented foods.

- Enjoy moderate- to high-energy workouts such as cycling, hiking, core workouts, HIIT, boxing, dancing, treadmill runs, elliptical sessions, and other cardio exercises.

- Sweat-inducing classes such as hot yoga and other heated workouts can also be satisfying in this phase.

- For maximum growth, trim your hair during the waxing moon.

Soul

- Start a new habit, hobby, workout, sport, or project if you are so inclined.

- If your energy feels scattered, try choosing one lifestyle area to focus on for this phase. It could be experimenting with intermittent fasting, trying a new fitness program, deep-diving into a new creative project, or researching ways to build wealth and invest.

- Connect with the earth by gardening, hiking, swimming in natural bodies of water, and other uplifting activities in nature.

Transitioning to the Next Phase

Energies are building and they will soon culminate in the peak of this cycle—a short window of time when we can practice experiencing life in full bloom. In this phase you did magical work to transform your ethereal heart and soul desires into living, breathing actions and habits. Like a Cycle Habits maven, you curated and designed a set of practices to support your success and wellness for many cycles to come. Keep practicing, aligning and realigning as needed.

If you've heard about the Law of Attraction or manifesting principle of "acting as if," you'll want to be ready to engage in it in this next phase, Thrive. In Thrive you will reach your peak of peachy ripeness and be ready to live the life of your dreams, even if only for a day. You'll taste the sweet nectar of your desires coming to fruition. Get ready to glow!

Chapter 6

THRIVE

• • • • • • • • •

> **Moon Phase:** Full Moon and Waning Gibbous Moon
> **Menstrual Phase:** Ovulation
> **Season:** Summer
> **Element:** Fire
> **Energetic Attribute:** Passion
> **Essence:** Vibrancy, vitality, peak, wholeness, perform, radiate, perfection, beauty, shine, confidence, abundance, intensity, celebrate, circulate, sensuous, glow, amplify, joy

The moment you've been waiting for—a mid-Summer day, the full bloom of a rose, the point of climax, the perfectly ripe peach, the peak of vitality and beauty, the moon at its fullest and brightest. You have arrived and are ready to Thrive! This is your moment to shine and experience the beauty of life at its fullest. Blink and you'll miss it. During this short phase, be sure to prioritize fun, passion, creativity, flow, and happiness. Here, you will live and embody your most joyful vibration.

When I moved to Los Angeles from London over a decade ago, ride-sharing companies weren't yet fully established, so there were no apps that let you simply click to book a ride. Instead, I spent my free time exploring the city by walking to destinations, catching rides with friends, or using traditional cab services. I hadn't really budgeted for a car since I was so used to walking or catching a bus or the tube (subway) in public-transport-friendly London. I figured that while I saved up for a car I would make do with walking or using cabs. This got old real quick! Imagine, if you will, a tall blonde dressed head-to-toe in European-style fashion (button-up blouse, pencil skirt, heels) on her way to work walking across a six-lane intersection with *no one else on foot around* while guys stared and whistled at her from their cars. Talk about intimidating. It was clear that I would need to magic up a car as soon as possible.

I turned to my go-to manifesting tools of affirmations and mantras, but also took it up a notch and engaged in acts of sharing. I donated to charities, volunteered to feed families in need on Thanksgiving, and helped friends out when they needed it, all the while imagining that the energy I was expending with my sharing actions was multiplying and in turn helping me to rise out of this place of lack that I had found myself in. It wasn't long before a friend proposed an offer that I couldn't refuse: She asked if I would drive her to the airport for an upcoming trip and pick her up when she returned a week later. In the meantime, I could use her car while she was away. At first I felt that this was too generous an offer and told her I was happy to drive her to the airport and pick her up, but I didn't need to use her car while she was away. She reassured me that it was fine and that it would make her happy to know that I would be using it, so I gratefully accepted. During that week I had the opportunity to "act as if" I had a car of my own. As I drove my friend's car to go grocery shopping, visit the beach, and cruise down Sunset Boulevard, I visualized this feeling of freedom being a natural part of my L.A. life. After I returned the car to my friend, I tried to revisit the feelings of happiness and freedom as often as possible in my everyday life. I followed my joy and began to put my attention toward things that I could do without a car and yet still stir up those good feelings.

I began to experiment with creating raw-food snacks and candies. Hours flew by as I blended, chopped, dehydrated, and decorated. The results were cookies, chocolates, macarons, and kale chips all made without heat using healthy ingredients like fruits, seeds, nuts, and cacao that when raw maintain their enzymes and nutrients. I loved playing with flavors and colors, using rose water and beet juice to create fragrant pink macarons and intricate candy molds to make raw chocolate truffles with pistachio filling. I got so good at it that I was producing small custom orders for friends and my healthy treats were being purchased as corporate holiday gifts, served at a fashion event, and even sold at a café in Hollywood. It all felt very exciting. I loved being able to create healthy foods that nourished and delighted people. The only problem was I had to rely on friends or rental cars to help me with delivery.

What was once a self-serving dream of owning a car for my own convenience and enjoyment took on a broader, more virtuous purpose—with a car I would be able to deliver my raw-food snacks to friends and stores all over town. I decided that I *absolutely* needed a car. It would help not only me, but also others. The next time I spoke with my dad I mentioned that I was starting a little side business making and selling raw-food snacks. He thought this was a great idea, and when I told him I was saving up to buy a car so I could deliver them around town, he offered to help me with a generous deposit. It just so happened that his next trip to visit me coincided with a Memorial Day sale at the dealership, and we got a great deal on a Toyota Prius. My dream had come to fruition, and although in the end the raw-food venture turned out to be more of a hobby than a thriving business (raw cookies take 12 hours to dehydrate), the car served me well for the next 10 years of my life, safely getting me to where I needed to go and enabling me to share quality time with friends and help them out when needed. By allowing myself to fully receive and enjoy the experience of driving a car around town, it brought my "future dream" into the present moment. This instantly removed any forces of resistance and lack. When I consistently followed my joy and imagined a greater purpose to my desire (to share with others), it elevated my vibration and unlocked the manifestation. You can apply this formula to your own life and the desires *you* wish to manifest by engaging with the exercises in this chapter, so let's get started by exploring the potent energy of the Thrive phase.

Lights, camera, action! The stage is set and it's time to take the lead in bringing your manifestation storyline to life. Full-moon energy beams down on you like a spotlight as you live in alignment with your desired manifestation. Behind the scenes, estrogen rises to the occasion, ensuring you have that superstar glow—thanks to a boost in collagen, confidence, and communication.

At the beginning of the cycle, the Attune phase, you worked on subconscious attraction, and here in the Thrive phase it's all about conscious embodiment—an outward expression of your inner desires. If Attune represents the potentiality of a dream, then Thrive is where it takes physical form. It's here. And if it's not quite here, then just go ahead and *act* as if it's here. Because even if your desire hasn't yet manifested IRL, there's plenty you can do to access the *feelings* that your manifestation will bring you, even in small ways.

During the Thrive phase we reach the peak of our cycle—ovulation, culminating in the release of an egg. Our bodies are primed for attraction and creation. The rising estrogen level can deliver shinier hair, increased collagen, and a sense of Venusian vitality. We're likely to feel more energized, articulate, and confident, naturally presenting our best selves to the world. Our brains undergo changes that can enhance communication skills, with estrogen boosting connectivity in areas linked to verbal fluency and social interaction. It's the opportune time to give a presentation, go on a date, pitch a concept, or do anything else that requires us to express ourselves with confidence and charisma.

Inherently linked to feminine energy, the moon is connected to receptivity, creation, and transformation. As the culmination of light in the night sky, the full moon can amplify our feelings and emotions. Astrologically, the full moon brings a sense of completion and sheds light on things that were previously hidden, making it a time of revelation.

Summer, the season with the most light, is also associated with the Thrive phase. It's a time of abundance, heightened energy, and outward expression. Warm Summer days boost serotonin production, evoking feelings of joy and playfulness. The Thrive phase is our hot girl Summer era.

On a metaphysical level, Fire is viewed as a powerful force of creation, destruction, and renewal. Intrinsically linked to the Thrive phase, Fire symbolizes the power to transform. It helps us burn away the old and step into new beginnings. Fire embodies the inner spark that motivates us to take bold action and follow our passions. It fuels ambition and creative drive, empowering us to move forward with purpose and enthusiasm. Its warmth creates inviting spaces for gathering, helping to shape social bonds and enhance our connections with others.

The Thrive phase is also linked to the energy of passion. When we allow ourselves to feel passionate about the things we wish to manifest, it ignites action and fuels creativity and expression, inspiring us to bring our dreams to life. Passion is inherently magnetic. By nurturing emotional resonance with our desires during this phase of amplified energy, we can help to draw them into our reality! During this phase you may feel unstoppable, so be mindful of what you commit to. Overcommitting to future plans may seem tempting, but energy levels are likely to dip as you progress through the two following cycle phases, so you may find yourself regretting having a packed schedule filled with obligations. Instead, maximize your vibrant energy by directing it toward activities you can do *right now* to manifest your most cherished desires and goals.

Where to Begin

The Attune and Thrive phases act as opposite energetic poles of a cycle, just like the new moon and full moon, and are relatively short (about three days) compared with the longer phases of Awaken (the follicular/waxing moon phase) and Surrender (the luteal/waning moon phase), which can be between one and two weeks long. Much like fruit, the best time to enjoy the Thrive phase is at its peak ripeness and culmination. This aligns with either the full moon or your time of ovulation if you're aligning with the menstrual cycle. Plan activities in preparation for this time because it's a brief window in which to draw your future wishes into the present moment.

If you are aligning with the moon cycle, use a moon cycle tracker (see "Resources" on page 264 for suggestions) and mark your schedule now for the next six months of new moons and full moons so you can be well prepared to take advantage of the Thrive phases. If you are aligning with your menstrual cycle, you may prefer to track this on more of a daily basis and approximate the time when you expect to ovulate one month at a time. There are several cycle tracking apps and websites available to help you keep track. (See "Resources.")

There are three exercises that flow in sequence to help you make the most of this short phase, followed by the "Thrive Phase Practices" section that includes additional practices and tools, any of which can be chosen for future revolutions though this phase so it never gets boring. For your very first journey through the Thrive phase, start with these three core exercises in order:

1. Act as If
2. Return to Joy
3. Expand Your Purpose

If you don't have time to complete this sequence of three exercises, that's perfectly okay. If you have to choose just one, do the Act as If exercise so you can consciously embody your desires coming to life during the powerful, expansive energy of this phase.

It's Time to Thrive!

This is an exciting phase in which you have the opportunity to activate your heart and soul desires by bringing them into the present moment through conscious embodiment. Begin the exercises within a day or two on either side of the full moon or your predicted time of ovulation.

. . . .

How Do I Know When I'm Ovulating?

With our busy lives, we may not even notice the signs of ovulation unless we are specifically looking for them.

Ovulation usually occurs sometime between days 12 and 17 of your menstrual cycle. For women with a 28-day cycle, ovulation usually happens around day 14, but this can vary. When you're ovulating, you might notice your cervical mucus becomes clear and sticky, similar to egg whites, and some women feel mild cramps or a little twinge in their lower abdomen. Your sex drive might kick up a notch, and your breasts could feel a bit more tender than usual. You may also have a keener sense of smell, feel a little bloated, or even experience a tiny bit of spotting. Your body temperature can go up slightly just after ovulation due to increased progesterone. You can track your body temperature first thing in the morning with a basal thermometer or wearable device synced with an app. By tracking your temperature over several cycles, you can see the shifts and better predict ovulation. If your cycle is irregular or if you are taking hormonal birth control, then you might opt to align with the moon cycle.

. . . .

1. Act as If

While it may be unrealistic to "act as if" your manifestations have already come to fruition all day every day, could you try it for just a day or two? Totally doable! That's your challenge in this Thrive phase: to physically drop into the sensation—and yes, delusion—of your wish having been fulfilled, and to fully experience those good-feeling vibes. Design an experience in which you physically participate in an activity that aligns with the way your desired manifestations would make you feel. The art of manifesting involves both inner work and outward action.

Get creative and plan something that will imbue you with these good feelings in the here and now. In this way, you are bringing your future into the present moment. So, let's get delulu, even if it's only for a few hours. Here are some examples:

Desire: To travel
Embodiment ideas: Go sightseeing close to home by visiting a place you've never been to before. This could be a nearby city, national park, museum, beach, famous restaurant, or other tourist destination. Take photos and share them with friends or family members and tell them about your day. Plan a mini staycation by clearing your schedule and taking time to relax. Visit a nearby resort or luxurious hotel for tea or a mocktail in the lobby. Immerse yourself in another culture by reading travel guides, watching shows, or researching ingredients for an authentic meal from that country.

Desire: To launch your own business
Embodiment ideas: Host a small get-together for friends and share a sample or sneak peak of what your business would offer. Prepare a brief PowerPoint presentation to introduce your idea. Visit local businesses to offer them a free or low-cost "lunch and learn" event where you can share a topical class with participants. Rent a fun dress and do a photoshoot with a friend or local photographer to promote yourself and your business. Record a video about a topic that's important to you and consider posting it on social media to promote your ideas and grow an audience.

Desire: To own a home
Embodiment ideas: Attend open houses in a nice area where you'd love to live, even if the prices are beyond your current budget. Visit inspiring home decor stores to compare the fixtures

and finishes and take notes on your favorite pieces or create an online mood board to capture decor and layout ideas for your ideal home. Write a list of who you'll invite to your housewarming dinner party, and think about what the menu will be.

Desire: To grow wealth
Embodiment ideas: Do some research and consider opening an investment account for making a small stock purchase from a company you like and watch its value grow. Attend online courses and watch videos about investing. Read some of the top 10 wealth and money books and take action on the ideas that resonate with and feel expansive to you. Place yourself among wealthy people by attending an interest group, sporting event, or networking group where entrepreneurs or people you admire socialize.

Desire: To be fit and healthy
Embodiment ideas: Sign up for a one-day pass at a gym you'd love to be a member of and spend the day enjoying the facilities, fitness classes, and equipment. Visit a fitness store and make a wish list of the items you'd like to own. Organize a walk with friends to a park or lake and make it fun by coordinating your outfits or stopping for a juice or healthy snack together afterward. Visit a discount store and spend around $20 on a cute clothing item, prop, or piece of equipment that you can use to work out at home.

Desire: To find love
Embodiment ideas: Create a Love List of the values and character traits you are looking for in a soulmate. Visit friends or family members who are happily married and let them know that you're open to love and ask what advice they might have

for you. Attend a speed-dating or meetup gathering to socialize with like-minded singles. Spend time with friends or family members who love you and make small handmade gifts or cards or special treats for them. Find a heart-centered guided meditation that you'd like to do daily.

Desire: To own a new car
Embodiment ideas: Book an appointment to take the car you'd love to own on a test drive and spend time at the dealership learning all about it. Rent the car of your dreams for a day or two and have fun driving it around and taking photos of it.

Now it's *your* turn! Write down one of your desires along with your embodiment ideas and schedule the time to act as if.

You may want to create an "Act as If" wish list of things you'd like to do each time the Thrive phase comes around so you can immerse yourself in uplifting activities that align with the feelings you wish to manifest.

2. Return to Joy

Your challenge is to find your way back into the high-vibe feelings of joy, happiness, peace, stability, or whatever good feeling it was that you practiced attaining during the Act as If exercise. We are focused on conscious embodiment and outward expression in this Thrive phase, which means you'll want to be *doing* things to help yourself return to your good feelings. By taking aligned action, your inner radio station will tune to a single frequency (feeling), resonating through your being for long enough to start attracting what you desire. When you find yourself out of alignment with your good-feeling vibes (because life happens), try journaling on these questions:

- What will it take to get myself into a better-feeling vibe?
- How can I revisit the good feelings I've recently experienced?
- What's a new or different way in which I can follow my joy today?
- In what ways can I express good feelings with others?
- How can I view a setback as a redirection?
- What am I passionate about?

Our energy is amplified during this brief Thrive phase, so whenever we shift into a space of appreciation and happiness, we radiate with a high vibration that can magnetize us to attract more of the same into our lives. Practice beginning with a small spark of joy over something you appreciate and then consciously expand it. Stay in your happy zone for as long as you can, and when you inevitably get distracted, resolve to return to joy again. Take it inch by inch, moment by moment. Challenge yourself to do this for 24 hours. Life sure can deal us some curveballs, and it can sometimes feel like a challenge to return to joy. Don't force it. Sit with your feelings, let them wash over you like a wave, learn from them, and then when it feels right, try to find just a tiny opening toward a better feeling and imagine it expanding from there.

3. Expand Your Purpose

When we follow our joy, magic can unfold, inspiring us to not only invest in ourselves but also expand our impact by thinking and acting in ways that benefit others. It can move us to feel a sense of purpose and enable us to share from our overflow without feeling burned out. By truly believing that the things we desire will create a positive ripple effect and touch lives beyond our own, we cultivate a deeper sense of worthiness in receiving them. The energies of expansion, excitement, purpose, and sharing help to attract our desired manifestations to us. In this exercise, we ask how our manifestations will benefit others and not just ourselves.

Exercise:

Write about the things you want to manifest and think of ways in which they could also benefit those around you. How could some of your desired manifestations help you to bring your best self to others, or even help others directly? Why is what you want a good thing? Write a convincing argument about why your manifestation will be of great benefit by having an expanded purpose beyond your own life.

Here are some examples:

Manifestation: A new home
Expanded purpose: To be a safe place for me to rest and replenish so I can give to others from my overflow. To have an opportunity to share my beautiful new home with others by hosting get-togethers to foster connections with family and friends. To be a space where I can create a positive environment that's conducive to personal growth, creativity, rest, and wellness. To be a space where I can properly care for my belongings and follow a healthy lifestyle, enabling me to share my positive energy with others.

Manifestation: Designer clothing and accessories
Expanded purpose: To enable me to look and feel stylish, confident, and professional so I can make a good impression in the

workplace or with clients to enhance my career opportunities in a way that helps me share my gifts and talents with the world. To enable me to donate items that I no longer need to people who can benefit from them. This creates an inspiring example for others who wish to invest in themselves, build wealth, feel confident, and manifest their desires.

Manifestation: Home gym equipment
Expanded purpose: To make it convenient for me to be healthy and active on a regular basis so I can bring my best energy and confidence to my career, family, and friends. To enable me to overcome limitations and excuses for not keeping active and become an example of wellness for my family and others. To help me reduce stress and get a better night's sleep so I can be more productive during the day. Owning my own equipment will allow me to share it with others who are also inspired to improve their wellness.

Now it's your turn! I bet you'll find that your desires are far from selfish. Take a few deep breaths, open your heart, and write down all the ways in which your manifestations can help create more light in the world around you.

The Moon Within

Humans have always lived under the glow of the moon, and its cycles have played a role in shaping our behaviors. Although modern life has distanced us from nature's rhythms, there's evidence that the moon still quietly influences us. These lingering patterns, known as circalunar rhythms, might be subtle, but they hint at how deeply connected we once were to the moon's phases. For our ancestors, the moon acted as a celestial guiding light. Luminous full moons lit up the darkness, making it easier to hunt, gather, and form connections. In contrast, the pitch-black nights of the new moon encouraged rest and safety, providing protection from predators. Coastal communities depended on the moon's pull on the tides to time fishing and foraging. Over countless generations, these rhythms became intertwined with human biology, shaping how we live, work, and rest. Researchers believe that in the days before artificial light, moonlight may have played a role in synchronizing ovulation among women in close-knit groups. This alignment could have helped communities work together to raise children and strengthened social bonds. Even today, there are signs that lunar phases might still influence reproductive hormones. One study found that women with menstrual cycles longer than 27 days may experience intermittent synchronization with the lunar cycle, particularly during phases of greater moonlight.[1] The moon can also affect our sleep. When the full moon brightens the night sky, it can suppress melatonin, the hormone that helps us wind down and fall asleep. This might explain why people tend to stay awake later and sleep less deeply during the full moon.[2]

Even though we've largely tuned out these natural rhythms with our brightly lit cities and busy schedules, the moon's quiet pull reminds us of the ways we're still connected to the natural world. Its cycles are woven into the fabric of our biology, offering a glimpse into how our ancestors lived in harmony with the ebb and flow of nature.

. . . .

Thrive Phase Practices

You're about to unlock the sacred codes to embodying your most radiant self—to becoming "that girl" with effortless feminine presence, illuminating any room you choose with your confidence, fierceness, and joie de vivre. Heart-centered, high-vibe, and unapologetically magnetic. Have fun with these goddess-worthy practices any time you're gliding through the Thrive phase, or whenever you feel called to.

Being Open to Receive

There's no time like the present to further explore the topic of feminine energy since we're in the phase aligned with ovulation and the glorious full moon, both of which are peak moments of receptivity and radiance. During ovulation, a woman's body is primed to receive, mirroring the full moon's luminous reflection of the sun's light, which symbolizes the union of feminine and masculine energies. The moon, representing the feminine, doesn't generate its own light, but instead reflects the sun's power, embodying a worthiness that comes from *being* rather than doing. Just as the moon reflects the sun without changing itself, as a feminine energy being, your value isn't something to be earned or proven—it's intrinsic and always present. This receptive energy contrasts with the action-driven need to "do" for validation. We can practice releasing the need to chase or force outcomes and instead experiment with attracting what aligns with us naturally. It's an invitation to trust that what is meant for us will come, as we align our desires with the cyclical flow of feminine energy. Know that you are inherently worthy of receiving good things in your life. We can desire all sorts of things, but if we don't truly feel like we are worthy of them, we may energetically push them away, or have hesitant energy where part of us desires the dream but part of us feels like it's too much, or undeserved, or not meant for us. Receiving good things is exciting in theory, yet it can often feel uncomfortable if you are more accustomed to taking matters into your own hands.

By being open to and curious about opportunities, you can avoid closing off potential channels of abundance. Your desired manifestations could arrive through another person serving as a conduit, if that happens to be the channel of least resistance. It could be a new person you meet who volunteers to connect you with someone who is looking to invest in exactly what you have to offer, a co-worker who wants to set you up on a blind date, or a loved one who offers to help you with something. The art of receiving gracefully can change the trajectory of your life. Allowing life's blessings, large and small, to reach you is a practice you want to nurture.

Many of us, myself included, have lived the majority of our lives in a way that is routinely aligned with our masculine energy, since this way of being is prevalent in today's culture. If that's also the case for you, the practice of receiving can feel quite healing to your mind, body, and spirit, as it has for me. Of course, there may be other subtle influences that can stand in the way of our ability to receive—our sense of pride, uncertainty about our worthiness, or concern that we'll owe someone something in the future. I invite you to gently notice the everyday moments when you can open yourself to receiving in ways that feel joyful and nourishing and observe any resistance that comes up. Here are some ways that you can practice the feminine art of receiving:

- Take compliments from others without deflecting them with humor or being self-deprecating. You can also let them know how it makes you feel (appreciated, happy, touched).

- Allow others to assist you if it feels safe to do so. When a friend, family member, or colleague offers to help you with something, be open to receiving their support. Accepting help from others sometimes requires us to acknowledge our vulnerability. This is a strength rather than a weakness, allowing us to form deeper friendships and connections. Consider embracing the opportunity to receive help instead of withdrawing from those who genuinely care.

- When you receive a gift or blessing in your life, take a moment to note how uplifting it feels. Pause and feel the sensations of receiving something wonderful.

- Be mindful of overgiving. When we provide excessive support or resources to others at the expense of our well-being, it can lead to burnout. Allow yourself the space to perform self-care.

- Explore affirmations that promote self-love and be aware of any harsh inner voices that may arise. When you notice these critical thoughts, remind yourself, "I am worthy of receiving beautiful gifts and blessings." This practice can help cultivate a kinder internal dialogue and reinforce your sense of worthiness.

- Practice being, rather than doing. Schedule time to rest and restore your energy, especially during the Attune and Surrender phases.

- In quiet times of meditation or prayer, ask to receive guidance, wisdom, love, healing, or blessings. Make a note of any messages or revelations you may receive.

- Consider that the gifts and blessings you receive originate from universal Source energy, flowing through the people, situations, and experiences in your life. What if giving and receiving, at its essence, is a collaborative partnership between you and the source of creation? Take a moment to reflect on and journal about this concept. How might acknowledging this connection resonate with you, and what insights might arise?

The Power of Presence

Often when we think about our desired manifestations, we view them as something we don't yet have. It can feel as if they are somewhere "over there" in the future, and yet here we are right here—in the present. This can create a sense of lack and perpetuate the energy of chasing our desires, but not necessarily reaching them.

Being fully present is one of the most powerful tools for attracting your desires, and there's no better time than the potent Thrive phase to engage with your desired feelings, right here and now. Because you're done with waiting and chasing, right? We often become attached to the past or future, but the present moment is where real change happens. By anchoring in "the now," you can make clear, conscious choices that align with your goals.

From a neuroscience perspective, being present activates the prefrontal cortex, the part of the brain involved in intentional thought, focus, and decision-making—which happens to be heightened during ovulation. When you're mindful and aware, your brain produces more gamma waves, which are associated with a higher level of cognition, greater clarity, and a stronger ability to hold a goal in mind. In a state of presence, you're better equipped to set clear intentions and pursue them without interference from old fears, doubts, or distractions.

Quantum physics suggests that focused attention and intention can influence reality at a subatomic level. The quantum observer effect posits that the act of observation can alter the behavior of particles, indicating that consciousness itself may play a role in shaping reality.[3] When you consciously focus on an intention while staying present, you might be more likely to "collapse" potential outcomes into the reality you desire, suggesting that our consciousness can indeed interact with the fabric of reality.

By drawing your attention to the present, you not only engage with the world more vividly but also align your mind with your goals. This alignment helps to reduce energy "leaks" that come from distractions or negative thought patterns. Being present can empower you to manifest your desires from a place of grounded intention and conscious choice.

Exercise:

Throughout the day, whenever you notice a distraction, write it down on a "distraction list" to revisit later, and get back to being in the present moment.

1. Note:

- What distracted me (e.g., phone notifications, random thoughts)
- When it occurred and how I felt (e.g., stressed, tired)
- Why I'm feeling drawn to this distraction right now (e.g., boredom, habit, the need for a break)

2. Reflection:

At the end of the day, review your list and ask:

- What were the most common distractions?
- How did each distraction impact my goals?

3. Empowerment:

Decide on some approaches you could take to:

- Reduce distractions
- Honor your body's need for breaks proactively taken to rest, hydrate, and nourish yourself
- Reenergize yourself about your goals

By bringing awareness to what is distracting us, understanding its impact on our thoughts and feelings, and exploring ways to return to the present moment, we practice intentionally attracting our dreams to us.

Create a Living Vision Board

Imagine walking around inside your very own 3D vision board, drawing your desires closer to yourself each day. I used this practice to manifest my dream of living near the beach. There were many weekends when I escaped the hectic pace of Los Angeles and headed to picturesque Malibu to enjoy the long stretches of sandy beaches. It took me over an hour to get there, and on Sunday evenings I would often be stuck in traffic for hours on the way home, along with everyone else who had flocked to the beach that day. Sometimes on my way to or from the beach I would take a little detour and drive around the neighborhoods of Malibu and Pacific Palisades to admire the coastal homes and apartments within reach of the sandy shore. I even crashed an open house or two and picked up a few design tips. The home decor in these beachfront neighborhoods used a lot of natural coastal hues of blue, seaglass green, sandy beige, and white. Little by little I transformed my L.A. apartment into a chic coastal home. I chose soft, muted blue curtains and cushions to go with my white furniture, added a small aquarium, placed a few small potted palm trees on my balcony, and displayed a collection of faux coral pieces on my bookshelf. It started to feel like I really was living close to the beach. I may even have drifted off to sleep a few times imagining that the distant hum of traffic on Robertson Boulevard was the sound of waves breaking on the shore.

A few months later, during a visit to a beautiful beach neighborhood in a nearby town, I popped into an open house and met my future husband. Today we live about a 10-minute drive from the beach and often spend our weekends walking along the shore and enjoying the ocean. Using the power of inescapable 3D visualization, I had brought the beach to me. I had stepped into the reality of living in a coastal home by transforming my then home into a living vision board. In this way, what I desired became something I already had, not something I was perpetually waiting for. There's a huge difference between the energy of expectation and the energy of waiting. The energy of waiting can hold a manifestation perpetually in a waiting room. When you create at least a small piece of what you ultimately want to experience, it brings the future into the present and you experience it now. No more waiting games. By adding a touch of magic to your existing home, even though it may not be your dream home, you come to love the place you're in a little more than you had before and also love the idea of manifesting a better place. This ushers in the energies of appreciation and expansion.

Living vision boards can be a powerful way to "act as if" and bring your future dreams into the present moment. It's one of my favorite creative, hands-on ways of manifesting. In fact, I'm known to have converted a small walk-in closet into a meditation room by adding mood lighting, a salt crystal lamp, a tiny stool, and a bookshelf for my collection of spiritual books. I once found some large, square, brightly colored, designer-looking silky scarves for $10 at a discount store and hand-sewed them into large, Hermes-style floor cushion covers that added a sophisticated boho vibe to my bedroom. I also converted a linen closet in a small hallway connecting my bedroom and bathroom into a Carrie Bradshaw–style walk-though accessory closet by removing the doors and defining the space with vibrant, large-scale floral wallpaper. I changed the light fixture to a mini chandelier, painted the shelves for a pop of color, and created stylish vignettes by topping stacks of fashion books and *Vogue* issues with my favorite heels, jewelry, clutch bags, and crystals. These living vision boards not only elevated the apartment into something that felt much more glamorous, but also helped me to manifest expanded versions of them in the home I now live in. This very fun and practical form of "acting as if" really works!

Exercise:

Can you identify a room, corner, or other space in your home that you could transform into a mini version of what you'd really love to manifest on a much larger scale? Perhaps you're dreaming of a home gym, cozy reading nook, wellness sanctuary, or dream closet? Many of the items I used to upgrade my space were affordable because I acquired them at discount stores, yard sales, or flea markets. It's amazing what you can do with a sample-sized can of paint, a few decor items, a new shelf, fabric offcuts, string lights, and some plants or crystals, so have fun getting crafty!

Cultivating Confidence

Although we may not feel confident all of the time, thanks to the energies available in the Thrive phase, we can use this time to strengthen our belief in ourselves. We can reflect on what we're good at and build on it, cycle after cycle, prompting us to think and act from a space of self-empowerment. This brings momentum to the unfolding of our desires and removes doubt and resistance, helping us to become better manifesters. I'm a big believer in investing in yourself so you can live a life of fulfillment and share with others from your full cup. Take this moment to invest in *yourself*. Select one or more of the activities in this exercise.

Celebrate!

Make a plan to celebrate one of your accomplishments. It may be a recent victory, or something you're proud of from your past that wasn't fully celebrated or appreciated at that time. Whatever it is, choose a way in which you can acknowledge your accomplishment. This could be by spending a day following your passions, hosting a dinner, writing yourself a letter, buying a frame to display a photo of yourself or a certificate you've earned, or setting aside an afternoon to indulge in some self-care or one of your favorite pastimes.

Gifts and Talents

When certain skills come easily to us, we often downplay them or even assume that everybody has these same gifts. We are all different and we all have unique gifts. What are some of your natural talents? Perhaps you are creative, or you can strike up a conversation with anyone you meet or solve a problem in a snap. Reflect on your natural talents, and make a list of what you do well.

Positive Self-Talk

Our internal voice narrates our lives from moment to moment, accompanying us throughout each and every day. It is therefore important that our inner voice speak to us kindly and compassionately. Often, our inner voice can take on a parental or overly critical tone. After all, it wants to keep us safe. The good news is that our inner voice is trainable—think of it like artificial intelligence. We can control, monitor, and set its algorithms. On a day of your choosing, make it your mission to become aware of your thoughts. If a critical or unpleasant thought arises, catch it and then affirm something more positive and supportive. Record on a notepad or in a notes app each time you were able to transform a critical message into positive self-talk.

Admirable Traits

Write down the names of three people whom you truly admire. Perhaps they have had a positive impact on humanity, shared their extraordinary talents in ways that uplift others, overcome the odds to become successful, or invented a new way to do something. For each of these three people, write down some of the traits and characteristics you know or imagine they must have to have accomplished what they have. Perhaps they have tenacity, integrity, courage, compassion, resilience, curiosity, humor, creativity, or something else. After you're done, look at the list of traits and circle the ones you have also recognized in yourself at one time or another. Take a moment to reflect on and appreciate your positive traits.

Body Love

- How can you take care of your physical wellness today?
- Is there something you can do to appreciate your body?
- How might you feel empowered in your body today?

Reflect on these questions and think of a self-care act or habit related to your body that you could do today.

Heart Opening

The heart possesses a powerful energetic frequency that extends beyond the body, affecting not only our own health but also the emotional states of those around us. Research from the HeartMath Institute highlights that the heart generates the strongest electromagnetic field of any organ. Heart energy can synchronize with that of others and facilitate communication and connection on a bioenergetic level. HeartMath's findings emphasize that the heart is not just a physical organ but also a vital source of intelligence that can enhance intuition and foster deeper connections with others.[4] Achieving heart coherence can help you to attract your desires by radiating a more stable and positive energy. This aligned emotional state creates a clearer intention, making it easier to focus on desires without the interference of negative emotions or stress. It also allows you to recognize and seize opportunities that align with your aspirations as the heart's electromagnetic field acts as a kind of energetic broadcast system that can influence what you attract into your life. The key is authenticity; the heart responds to genuine emotions, not just positive thinking. Preliminary research has highlighted the heart's intuitive abilities—being able to respond to future events before they occur—suggesting that it plays a role in guidance and manifestation.

The heart chakra, known as *anahata* in Sanskrit, is a vital energy center that embodies love, compassion, and emotional connection. The heart chakra acts as a link, integrating the energies of the lower chakras, which relate to survival and emotions, with those of the upper chakras, associated with higher consciousness and intuition. When balanced, the heart chakra fosters healthy relationships, empathy, and a sense of belonging. It encourages openness, allowing the circuitry of love to flow.

When we cultivate heart-centered practices, we enhance our capacity for empathy, creating a ripple effect that positively influences our relationships and environments, ultimately leading to a more harmonious life. To align with and expand your powerful heart energy, try incorporating one or more of the following practices into your routine.

Heart-Opening Yoga

Perform yoga poses designed to open the heart chakra, such as Cobra Pose, Camel Pose, and Bridge Pose. These poses help release tension in the chest and shoulders while promoting emotional release and self-love. Regular practice not only enhances physical flexibility, but also fosters emotional resilience.

Acts of Sharing and Kindness

Acts of kindness allow you to share your love and compassion with others. They can be as simple as volunteering, sending a heartfelt note, or donating to a cause you care about. Acts of sharing cultivate a sense of community and connection, reinforcing the heart chakra's energy and supercharging your manifestations.

Heart Chakra Visualization

Practice heart chakra meditations that focus on breathing into the heart center. Visualize a green light (the color associated with the heart chakra) that expands with each breath, filling your body with love and compassion. You can also visualize channeling this energy to others, nurturing deeper connections.

Rose Quartz Heart Chakra Activation

Sit comfortably and hold a rose quartz crystal in your left hand. Place your right hand gently over your heart and set the intention "I allow love to flow freely in and out of my heart." Close your eyes and take three slow, deep breaths. With each inhalation, imagine a soft pink light—the energy of the rose quartz—entering your heart chakra. Visualize a warm, pink light glowing in the center of your chest and expanding with each breath. Feel it radiating compassion, love, and peace throughout your body.

Heartbeat Synchronization

Sit or lie down in a comfortable position and begin by taking a few deep breaths, allowing your body to relax with each exhale. Notice the rhythm of your heartbeat—this can be felt in your chest, neck, or wrist. Inhale deeply to the count of four, hold your breath for a count of four, and exhale slowly to a count of four. As you breathe, try to feel your heartbeat synchronize with your breathing. Inhale for four beats, hold for four, and exhale for four beats. Practice this synchronized breathing for up to five minutes. This technique uses the body's natural rhythms to create a sense of love and presence.

- -

The Five-Second Appreciation Tool

Diverting small irritations directly into appreciation before they can take hold can help us to rewire our thoughts into something positive instead of spiraling downward. When an irritating thought emerges, don't give it your attention. Train your mind to stop, count to five, and think of something you appreciate instead. In this way, you'll disrupt the process of dwelling on any feelings of frustration and lack. When confronted by negativity, our minds often go into problem-solving mode, but it isn't always constructive. It can easily lead to worst-case-scenario thinking. Intrusive thoughts can feel a lot like back-and-forth chatter, doubts, illogical fears, and what-if questions. Practice identifying these patterns of thinking as they emerge and quickly disrupting them with a better-feeling thought. Let's welcome appreciation as a magnet for more goodness and an antidote for feelings of lack.

Summon Your Fire

Whether it's the assertive bump of testosterone we receive during the Thrive phase or the brilliant boldness of the full moon, our feminine nature is infused with a powerful burst of fierceness during this time. I liken this energy to that of the planet Mars, a cosmic warrior and ruler of the astrological signs of Aries, known for forging new paths and creating breakthroughs, and Scorpio, marked by intensity and passion. And just like the courageous sword-wielding goddess Kali, we can draw upon this fierceness to slice through illusions and reveal the truth, create transformation, and move beyond our perceived limitations. This fire can be ignited through passion and creativity or sheer will and focus. If the density of pain and sadness needs to be destroyed in favor of a better life, or an outdated perspective needs to be shattered into a million pieces so we can never return to that way of being again, then this is the energy we want to summon.

In my teens I spent a lot of time locked away in my bedroom wishing for a different reality. There was family turmoil, divorce, and a longing for a mother's love that always eluded me. There was deep hurt. I spent many evenings listening to loud music on my headphones and purging my grievances onto the pink-lined pages of my secret diary. I was angry. At times I felt overlooked and unloved. I longed for a future where my essence and gifts were appreciated. I began to channel this intensity into art. I put pencil to paper and started to draw. At the time, I was listening to a lot of Guns N' Roses, so I decided to create a portrait of the guitarist Slash. I replayed the guitar solo from "Sweet Child O' Mine" over and over, inviting it to fuel me in drawing the most realistic, striking portrait I could possibly create. I wanted people to gasp when they saw it. I worked on this portrait night after night, shading and outlining each tiny detail, from the deep coil of strands within a lock of hair (of which there were many) to the delicate glistening rim of a tear duct. I wasn't just drawing with as much skill as I could muster, I was intentionally *channeling* all my emotions into the artwork. I didn't know it then, but I was alchemizing pain and difficult truths into something equally astonishing, but in a creative, passionate, elevated form. As I drew, I imagined that all this pain that I didn't know what to do with was being transformed by the creative process into something that would carry a brighter energy and bring me happiness someday. Somewhere deep inside me I just *knew* that there must be a light at the end of the tunnel. After I finished the portrait of Slash, it received the gasps of admiration and disbelief from friends that I'd hoped for.

I went on to pursue more creative outlets, expressing myself through photography, writing, fashion, and music. A few years later I had left home and forged my own path working in the music industry. I enjoyed seeing bands perform live and being involved in music management, promotion, and marketing, working for record labels and concert producers. One night Guns N' Roses was in town and I found out I would have the opportunity to meet the band backstage. I dug out my portrait of Slash, which had been filed away over the years, and brought it with me. As the gig was about to start, Slash and his bandmates were making their way from their tour bus to the back door of the venue in a hurry, passing by a long line of eager fans waiting to get their items autographed, but there was no time for signatures. As Slash entered the venue and walked by me to take the stage, I flashed him the portrait, and he stopped in his tracks, smiled, and signed it. He asked me if I'd drawn it and told me it was incredible. This felt like a full-circle moment. I remembered the hours spent in my childhood bedroom, sitting at my desk and drawing under the fluorescent lamp, listening to music and trying to escape the heaviness of my feelings. Somehow I had transmuted and reimagined that pain and angst into a fierce desire for more. A desire for a day when I would be happy and doing what I loved to do, and in time that's exactly what happened.

As feminine energy beings, we can be viewed in a certain way by society, and even view *ourselves* a certain way, perhaps feeling that we *always* have to be "nice" and not burden others with our feelings, and in the process it becomes second nature for us to dampen our difficult emotions. By courageously facing our emotions and transmuting them through creativity, we can release their heaviness and open ourselves up to new possibilities.

Exercise:

During the intensity of the Thrive phase, if you dare, summon your inner fire and fierceness to transform pain into passion. Reflect on what you may be numbing, denying, or ignoring. The challenge here is to transmute those intense or heavy feelings into a thing of beauty. Express yourself through a creative channel like art, music, crafts, photography, drawing, writing, painting, dance, or something else you feel called to do. Create with passion!

Full-Moon Charging

She's here! The beautiful and dazzling full moon, filling up the sky with light. Receive her magnificence by engaging in one of these full-moon charging practices in this cycle, or in a future one.

Crystals

Under the light of the full moon is a perfect time to charge crystals. Place your crystals in a safe spot outdoors on a clean dish just before or on the night of the full moon. If it's cloudy, that's fine; it will not affect the moon's energy charging. You can also put them on a windowsill, or even directly on the soil for grounding while they are being imbued with the moon's energy. When you bring them back inside the next morning, also charge them with your own intentions, and how you wish for them to support you in manifesting your heart and soul desires. While looking at the crystals, recite your intentions aloud if possible. Give thanks to the moon for charging and cleansing your crystals.

Moon Water

To create moon water, first check whether the upcoming full moon is an eclipse or not. If it is an eclipse, skip the moon water exercise until a non-eclipse full moon arrives. Choose a clean jar with a lid, such as a mason jar. Fill your container with filtered or spring water and infuse it with your intentions. Think of your desired manifestations and feel into the reality of having them come to fruition. Take a deep breath and dwell in your good-feeling emotions. Look at your jar of water and visually send your good-feeling vibes and intentions into the water and imagine it glowing with light. Place your jar outside in the moonlight, or on a windowsill. Collect it the next morning and use it as drinking water, for tea, as a room-cleansing spritz with essential oils, added to bathwater, or for your beauty and wellness routine.

Jewelry

The full moon is a wonderful time to cleanse and energize your jewelry, especially pieces you wear often. Consider including a bracelet you wear on your left wrist, which is symbolic of your feminine energy. The left side of the body is associated with receiving and intuition—qualities connected to the Divine feminine. By placing your jewelry under the nurturing glow of the full moon, you imbue it with gentle, feminine energy. Lay your jewelry on a clean dish or cloth and place it outdoors or on a windowsill where it can bathe in the moonlight. Before wearing your charged jewelry, hold it in your hands and set an intention for how you want your jewelry to serve as a reminder of your inner strength, beauty, and connection to the feminine. Recite your intention aloud if it feels right to do so and thank the moon for infusing your treasures with her energy.

Journal

Your journal is a sacred container for your inner work, desires, intentions, and affirmations. Find a comfortable space to sit (indoors or outdoors) under the light of the full moon and take a few moments to recharge and bless your journal energetically. Use this time to write affirmations, manifestation lists, or thoughts that align with your Heart and Soul Desires. Before writing, hold your journal and set an intention for the clarity and creativity you wish to flow through it. Reflect on the words it already holds—the lessons captured within its pages, and how they have guided your growth. Imagine the moon's light amplifying your journal's energy, empowering it to capture your dreams and inspire your next steps. Thank the moon for her illuminating energy and place your journal on a windowsill or outdoors in the moonlight overnight.

The Thrive Lifestyle

Prepare to Thrive with these lifestyle tips to support this high-vibe phase.

Mind

- Diffuse essential oils that support confidence and boost happiness, such as grapefruit, bergamot, sandalwood, and jasmine.
- Socialize, give presentations, make speeches, record videos, be the life of the party.
- Make room in your schedule to celebrate and have fun. Bend the rules, lighten your load, and take some me time.

Body

- Enjoy the highest-quality or your most loved meals during this brief window of time.
- Wear your favorite outfits that bring you the most confidence. Choose happy, bright colors if you feel inspired to. Bring out your special-occasion items such as designer-label shoes, matching lingerie sets, and leather accessories. Anoint yourself with high-quality perfume.

- Indulge in a spa session, mani-pedi, or hair appointment so you can look and feel your best and shine.

- Enjoy moderate to high-energy workouts. Consider trying those with a theatrical, sensual, or creative flair, or ones that are fun or new to you, such as dancing, ballet-barre routines, aerial yoga, a spinning class with mood lighting and high-vibe beats, skiing, sailing, or water sports.

- Style your hair and wear it in your favorite, most alluring way, or try a sexy new style. Embellish your look with sparkling, high-quality, or bold accessories. Have fun with makeup, wear eyelash extensions or more dramatic colors than usual, or give a glittery touch to your eyes.

Soul

- Practice being present as much as possible. Be, and feel into the present moment. Breathe deeply and bring your attention to your five senses and fully experience what you are seeing, hearing, smelling, touching, and tasting.

- Engage in activities and with people who help you feel uplifted and happy.

- Allow yourself the freedom to be creative, partake in high-vibe pursuits, and express yourself fully during the Thrive phase.

Transitioning to the Next Phase

Just as the moon's light gently retracts after she's illuminated the night sky, we too can take a step back from the spotlight and prepare for some much-needed rest and reflection as we enter the Surrender phase. As cyclical feminine energy beings we are not designed to operate at our peak energetic level at all times. Following the productive Awaken phase and burst of Thrive phase excitement, you're due for some cozy quiet time to spend on self-care and restorative practices. There'll be plenty of time to explore your inner world, mind-body connection, and emotional terrain, all while picking up a few tips on how to leverage your natural rhythms to support your manifesting journey while also conserving precious energy. It's time to plant your feet on the ground, take a breath, and assess where you are.

Chapter 7

SURRENDER

• • • • • • • • • • •

Moon Phase: Waning Gibbous, Last Quarter, and Waning Crescent
Menstrual Phase: Luteal (Premenstrual)
Season: Fall/Autumn
Element: Earth
Energetic Attribute: Grounded
Essence: Reflect, discern, release, observe, recognize, evaluate, thoughtful, identify, aware, appreciate, finalize, disengage, liberate, trust, healing, epiphany, harvest, truth, allow

Having put forth your high-vibe intentions during the Thrive phase, trust that more good things are on the way. Earthly and grounded, the Surrender phase is all about laying low, being practical, letting go, and allowing the best outcome to occur. In contrast to the Thrive phase, in this phase we tend to not want to draw attention to ourselves. It's a time to practice trust by releasing attachments, yet holding true to your innermost desires. Surrendering doesn't mean relinquishing a heartfelt dream. It's about releasing distractions and noise to focus on what truly matters: exploring your uniqueness and becoming deeply aligned with the vision you feel called to bring to life. To be in tune with this phase, let go of what you think you need and accept what shall be—for your highest good.

Coaching client Amelia's dream was to find love with a trustworthy, dependable guy who could also make her laugh and keep up with her spontaneous nature. She'd taken a break from dating apps after experiencing her fair share of lackluster dates. "Honestly, I'm feeling pretty jaded about dating," she confessed at our first coaching session. Amelia was compassionate, vibrant, driven, and fun. Her love for animals had led her to launch her own business—a mobile dog grooming service. One of her regular customers, Ryan, had recently asked her out on a date, but she hadn't committed to any plans yet. When I asked her why, she told me that she'd been busy at work. When I dug a little deeper it turned out that although Ryan seemed like a nice enough guy, he wasn't her usual type, and she was "still kind of hung up" on her ex-boyfriend, Julian. Amelia confided that something Julian had said when they broke up had stayed with her. He'd told her that no matter what he did, he felt like he couldn't make her happy. She'd been reflecting on this statement a lot and wanted some guidance in exploring why the relationship went off track and how she could start attracting a fulfilling long-term partnership.

Prior to Julian, Amelia had gone through several heartbreaks, and they all seemed to follow a similar pattern—starting out great, followed by a feeling of distance and disconnection a few months later. In some cases Amelia had attempted to fight for the relationship by putting more effort into fixing issues she thought could be contributing to the disconnection, but she often ended up feeling taken for granted or disrespected. We started exploring some inner-work exercises together, and

Amelia realized that in past relationships she had allowed herself to be treated in ways that she wasn't happy with for fear of going through another breakup. After some soul-searching, she transformed a long list of relationship grievances into a list of relationship desires.

Amelia wanted her next partnership to feel much more stable, caring, and connected. And although it made her feel vulnerable to admit it, deep down she wanted marriage. With this new clarity of desire in mind, she worked through some practices to help her forgive and release her past relationship hurts. Amelia also worked on self-forgiveness for allowing herself to be treated in ways that she regretted, and for continuing to pursue certain men when she wasn't happy with how they were showing up for her. She also came up with a set of new boundaries to embody going forward.

While Amelia was undertaking this inner-work journey, Ryan was reaching out occasionally by phone or text and they'd had some enjoyable conversations. Amelia was warming up to him. When she mentioned that he'd recently dropped in to see her to give her a little gift I asked her what it was. "I don't know, I couldn't accept it," Amelia told me. She found it difficult to put into words why she felt that she couldn't accept Ryan's gift. She was curious about it, she thought it was a sweet gesture, and she definitely liked him. I asked her if she found it uncomfortable to receive things from people—gifts, help, advice, compliments. She thought for a moment and said, "Well, he did also offer to help me carry some heavy boxes into my van the other day, but I didn't want him to go to any trouble, and besides I can move heavy boxes on my own." She paused and smiled, "So yes, I guess you could say I do feel uncomfortable with receiving." After taking time to reflect on what was preventing her from accepting help or kind gestures from others, Amelia realized that she felt more in control when things were happening on her own terms.

She also realized that by rejecting offers of kindness, she was energetically pushing people away, even though deep down she craved connection. Over the next few weeks Amelia practiced receiving kind gestures from others that felt sincere and safe to receive. Things with Ryan continued to go well, and she told me that she had accepted his gift—a sterling silver name tag for her dog, Max, in the shape of a bone. She and Ryan both owned dogs called Max, and he'd thought it would be a fun gift.

Late one evening I received a text from Amelia stating, "Julian's back!" followed by, "He wants to know if he can come over now and talk. What should I say?" I suggested that Amelia take some time to calmly revisit her list of boundaries about how she wanted to be treated, think about what kind of response felt good to her, and consider when the right time would be to respond to her ex-boyfriend. The next time we met, Amelia and I talked more about embodying boundaries. It's the difference between *telling* someone not to text you to meet up late at night versus *embodying* your boundary on an energetic level and making that inner decision and commitment to yourself about what you are or are not available for. In Amelia's case, she'd decided that she didn't want to put herself in a position of having her ex-boyfriend come to her house late at night, plus she was unwinding after a busy week and halfway through a captivating novel. She decided that there was no need to respond right away or allow his text to spark anxiety, so she calmly waited until the next morning to respond in a pleasant way about meeting up for a coffee sometime to talk. She honored her boundary by physically not replying to the late-night request to meet up. She responded at a time that suited her and in a way that wasn't charged with emotion. In relationships (including friendships), we can practice expressing our boundaries in a grounded way, even if we have to repeat them sometimes. I shared with Amelia that by embodying our boundaries, it energetically teaches people how to respond to us through our actions and overall vibe. "Oh, I get it, it's like training people on how to treat you. I know *all* about training!" she said. Whether it's the person we date, friends, family members, or co-workers, people can sense our vibe in a way that's similar to how our furry friends pick up on their trainer's energy. We are in charge of our own vibration, decisions, and what we allow. When we embody the energy of a person who places importance on what she gives her time and attention to, people pick up on it without many (or any) words needing to be said. That's the power of embodiment.

Over the course of the next few months, and with the help of Ryan and Julian, Amelia was able to practice receiving gestures that felt good to her, embodying her boundaries of how she wanted to be treated, overcoming anxiety around connecting with others, honoring her needs, relinquishing the urge to overgive or fix things, and surrendering to her heart's desire for a long-term committed relationship. In time, Amelia opened herself up to the love, stability, and devotion that Ryan offered her, and they became engaged. She was able to make inner shifts that were reflected and rewarded in her external reality. We all carry with us emotional hurts from the past and blind spots in how we may be hindering the manifestation of our desires. I invite you to use the inner-work tools and exercises in this chapter to spark self-inquiry, transform dissatisfaction into desire, and release unwanted baggage to create space for beautiful new things to manifest in your life.

Are You Ready to Surrender?

As we are summoned toward a more restful state, thanks to the release of the calm-inducing hormone progesterone during the luteal (premenstrual) phase, or the depletion of the moon's light as it wanes, it's an invitation to reflect and release. Both the hormonal shifts and the waning moon encourage introspection and completion—it's an ideal time for tidying up tasks, reflecting on goals, getting organized, letting go of what's unnecessary, and tuning in to our needs.

The energy of Fall, or Autumn, linked to this Surrender phase is a time of transition. Just as nature shifts—trees shed leaves to conserve energy for Winter, some animals prepare for hibernation, and daylight shortens—the season encourages internal change. This energy of "letting go" inspires us to shed unhelpful patterns and thoughts. It's also a time of harvesting, when we can gather insights and clues. Have you noticed any evidence of what you desire already emerging? Perhaps you see hints of it showing up in your life in small ways, or even in the lives of people you know. This can be a great sign that your desired manifestation is moving closer into your reality.

The Surrender phase is also connected to the element of Earth, which in spiritual traditions signifies a sense of security, nurturing, material wealth, practicality, and stability. This supportive energy inspires a realistic and sensible approach to life's challenges, helping us with decision-making. Earth energy reinforces the importance of conserving resources, making this an ideal time to shift into more nurturing and restorative activities, a diet of nourishing foods, and stress-reducing practices.

The energetic attribute of the Surrender phase is one of being grounded. When we feel grounded, we are better equipped to manage our emotions (which can be heightened at this time) and respond thoughtfully rather than react impulsively. Grounding energy invites us to make mindful adjustments to stay balanced and centered, fostering emotional resilience. Groundedness provides a sense of stability amid chaos or uncertainty. As we align with the energy of the Surrender phase, we have the opportunity to create a bridge between our intangible desires and their physical manifestation. Establishing this flow between thought and reality requires trust and surrendering the need to know how and when our desired manifestations will arrive. Preparing for our manifestations may involve decluttering and organizing, emotional release, or symbolically clearing space for new possibilities. View this phase as an opportunity for evaluation and recalibration—a time to assess whether your current actions align with your desired manifestations. The exercises and tools in this chapter will help you balance intention with physical action, cultivating the grounded readiness needed to welcome your desires into reality. Are you ready to embody trust in the midst of uncertainty?

Where to Begin

If you have a natural menstrual cycle and are not currently using a hormonal contraceptive, the best time to begin will be a day or two after ovulation, which could align with the second half of your cycle. If you are aligning with the moon cycle, you can begin after the full moon.

There are two exercises that flow in sequence to help you make the most of this phase, followed by a section called "Surrender Phase Practices" that is filled with additional, optional practices and tools that you might want to explore in future cycles. For your very first journey into the Surrender phase, start with these two core exercises:

1. Release and Reclaim
2. Embody Your Boundaries

They will assist you in releasing energetic debris and creating the foundation to protect your energy. If you aren't able to complete this sequence of two exercises, that's perfectly okay. You can choose any exercise that you are drawn to from the full selection of options in this chapter.

It's Time to Surrender

Have you taken bold actions toward manifesting your dreams over the previous phases of this cycle? Take a moment to feel proud of all that you have accomplished, trusting that every intention and action you have put forth will compound into blessings and gains as you continue working with natural energy cycles. The next two exercises offer you the opportunity to undertake powerful inner work to release any barriers that may be preventing you from receiving your heart and soul desires.

1. Release and Reclaim

During my studies to become a certified Law of Attraction practitioner, instructor Dr. Joe Vitale emphasized the role of forgiveness as a vital piece in the process of manifesting desires. He believes that by letting go of blame and embracing forgiveness we can open ourselves up to attracting our desires. Forgiveness for others and self-forgiveness allow us to experience a positive shift in our external reality by changing our inner state.

An unwillingness to forgive another person for something that happened in the past becomes an energetic obstacle in our present lives. Dense energetic baggage like anger, judgment, and resentment can create a metaphysical gate that blocks our ability to manifest desires. For this reason, we want to let go of this baggage and become a clear channel and energetic match to the good-feeling desires and feelings we wish to attract. By working on forgiveness and letting go of past judgments, we lighten our emotional load and elevate our vibration. I believe that part of the reason we are here in this world is to learn lessons of love and forgiveness with each other during our soul's journey. Forgiveness is not about letting the other person off the hook; its purpose is for self-healing through mental and emotional freedom. As Dr. Vitale teaches, "Modern society is rarely a forgiving society. From childhood, we have been taught that good deeds are rewarded while bad deeds are punished. There is no real middle ground." If we have gone years or even decades holding on to past hurts, it's time to let them go. Here's a practice I created to help you not only release the weight of past hurts but also reclaim the mental and emotional resources you've expended, allowing your precious energy to return to you—and *multiply* through your alignment with natural cycles!

1. Create a quiet, peaceful environment where you can be undisturbed for at least 20 minutes. Sit down comfortably with a notepad and pen nearby.

2. Close your eyes and imagine a mirror in front of you. Visualize the person you need to forgive reflected back to you from the mirror.

3. Notice what emotions surface as you observe them through this mirror. Do you feel any tension in your body? How has holding on to these emotions affected you?

4. Open your eyes and write a letter to the person in the mirror, without any intention to send it. Address each feeling honestly, expressing any hurt, frustration, or disappointment. Now, shift your focus and write about what you have learned or gained from this exercise, even if it's something small. For example, it could be resilience, patience, or clarity about your needs.

5. Hold the letter in both hands, close your eyes, and imagine yourself reclaiming the energy you've expended in having strong feeling about the person or situation. Visualize this energy returning to you in a stream of warm light, filling any spaces within you that feel empty, tense, or drained.

6. When you're ready, tear up the letter and affirm, "*I release you from this role in my life and reclaim my energy for my own growth and peace.*"

7. Take three deep breaths, letting each exhalation carry away any lingering tension. In your heart, visualize warmth and light, affirming "*I am free, and I allow peace to fill me.*"

Return to this practice as often as needed to let go of density and reclaim your authentic energy. This creates space for a renewed sense of peace and purpose so you can attract your desired manifestations with less friction in the way.

2. Embody Your Boundaries

"Nice girls finish last, sweetheart"—the taunting statement from my bestie Toby echoed over the car speakerphone as I frantically drove across town from one Target store to another trying to locate a limited-edition Missoni for Target espresso set for a mutual friend on my only day off that week. "It's rare!" I countered, "and she's not feeling great." I had promised her I would track it down, but despite visiting five stores and calling three others, I still couldn't find it anywhere. I wondered aloud whether I should give her the one that I had ordered. "Oh, girl, the one you set your alarm for to buy online at six A.M. while our friend sleeps in so she can go out later tonight?" teased Toby. I don't know if that was true, but I knew that this fruitless quest was chewing up my whole day and I was really feeling drained.

Looking back now, it's easy to recognize the pattern I was stuck in for many years—not wanting to disappoint people. Couple that with having a lack of clarity about my personal goals and desires and a fear of speaking up, it's no wonder I routinely felt overstretched. Conquer the occasional near-impossible task on behalf of others? Sign me up. Not speaking up about my needs until I fell ill with health issues? Hello, hormone imbalance. Being a girl without a strong sense of direction and not in touch with my true needs and desires, I had no clue about setting boundaries (doing that just sounded rude), and it kept me treading water for years. I had to learn to express myself and not be scared that my life would be rocked by the consequences. I learned that having boundaries not only helps protect your precious energy, it's also actually attractive to others. Eventually I learned to protect my time and energy. I prioritized healing, said no to certain invitations, turned down a few side jobs, and ended a friendship. I had to do what was best for my wellness.

Now I've made up for lost time, and I feel good about and worthy of protecting my energy so I can do things that elevate my life and the lives of others in a *much* broader way. It turns out that there is such a thing as being too "nice." Especially when we trample over our own needs, intuitive signals, enjoyment, and rest. Want to help others? Know your boundaries so you can become an effective, empowered woman who rises in life and inspires the same in all who witness her light.

Now that you've journeyed through all four phases of the cycle, you're likely getting a feel for how *you* want to direct your energy so it's being used to attract and magnify your desires. There will be ways in which you directed your energy in the past that you will no longer want to pursue—like getting involved in drama, arguments, unnecessary tasks, and other energy leaks. This is where boundaries can help. The way society often views boundaries is like lines drawn in the sand, marking the border another person should not cross in order to respect our energy. We can set boundaries with anyone who will listen, but unfortunately there's no guarantee they will keep to their side of the boundary line. I invite you to think about boundaries differently—as internal, energetic decisions that we decide upon, embody, and emanate. If we no longer want to waste our energy on arguments that go around in circles, we don't need to explain that decision to anyone, we can simply decide it (commit to yourself), embody it (physically leave the room or don't engage), and emanate it (act in ways that respect your own and others' energies).

In this workshop you'll first identify some of your boundaries and then activate your embodiment of those boundaries. This will help protect your life-force energy so when you *do* feel moved to help others, share with friends, do favors, and volunteer your time, you'll show up with your best, most attractive energy, feeling confident, renewed, and with a full cup, able to give from your overflow. That truly is the best way to help others.

Grab your journal and follow these steps to create and embody your boundaries:

Identify Your Boundaries

With intention, we can draw upon the energy of the Surrender phase to assist us in seeing where we need to create boundaries around our time and attention. Choose three or more of these journal prompts to reflect on where your energy and well-being may need protection and to decide on a boundary you would like to embody.

Reflection: Take note of relationships or interactions that tend to leave you feeling drained, taken for granted, resentful, overwhelmed, disrespected, or unsettled.
Boundary: In what ways could you protect your energy in scenarios like this? For example, if social gatherings or work demands feel exhausting, consider setting limits on your availability.

Reflection: Reflect on your Cycle Magic work over the previous two phases and bring to mind the desires and goals that matter most to you. What kinds of things would you like to make more time for in your life? For example, you might desire to carve out more time for self-care, family, career goals, or spirituality.
Boundary: What would you need to spend less time on to let yourself channel more time into achieving your desires and goals? For example, you might set a boundary limiting how much screen time you allow yourself each day.

Reflection: Do you regularly find yourself agreeing to things you later regret having to do?
Boundary: What kinds of things could you say no to or delegate to others? For example, you may have fallen into the habit of saying yes to a particular person regardless of how inconvenient their requests may be.

Reflection: Are there times when you feel obligated to respond to someone's request as soon as possible even though the situation is not urgent?
Boundary: In what ways could you set a boundary around communication to prevent burnout? For example, you might like to set a rule to not respond immediately to non-urgent requests.

Reflection: Bring to mind a situation where you felt physical tension, fatigue, or anxiety.

Boundary: What type of boundary could you put in place to provide yourself with more comfort? For example, before saying yes to invitations to join physically demanding workout classes you might want to check which menstrual cycle phase you'll be in.

Reflection: Recall a time when you overextended yourself to accommodate others at the expense of your well-being.

Boundary: Acknowledge it when you're giving too much and place boundaries that will maintain mutual respect. For example, you might want to reserve one day a week that is free of any scheduled plans.

Creating boundaries in these areas can help you protect your energy and prioritize what's most important to you. Boundaries can be flexible, so you may want to review and adjust them over time as your needs and relationships evolve.

Embodiment Practice

When you embody boundaries, your physical presence, actions, expressions, and energy project a quiet strength that communicates your limits to others intuitively. This helps you avoid having to overexplain or defend your boundaries because your energy reflects your inner conviction, which is often clearer than words alone. It's about fostering inner clarity on what you're willing to accept and what aligns with your well-being, which then translates naturally into action.

Exercise:

For each boundary that you identified in the previous exercise, write ideas on how you could begin to embody them.

Example:

Boundary: Not being in a car with someone who drives in a dangerous way

Embodiment: Drive myself, use a ride-share service or taxi, or take public transportation when meeting them. Take a credit card and a fully charged phone with me whenever I go out in case I have to order a ride unexpectedly. My safety is a priority.

Example:

Boundary: I need one hour to study at least three nights a week for a course I'm taking.

Embodiment: Use time blocking and set a reminder in my calendar. Switch phone and desktop notifications off during this time, and don't answer any messages. Create an environment conducive to studying by playing music that enhances focus or wearing noise-canceling headphones. Don't commit to plans during study time. Schedule study time for early enough at night that I don't get too tired for it. Politely decline invitations that conflict with study time and let the people I live with know in advance when I'll be studying.

Embodiment Activation

If you need an extra boost to really embrace and embody your new boundaries, try this embodiment activation on for size. From your list of boundaries, choose one that you'd like to begin embodying and follow the steps below. Repeat this practice for each new boundary you'd like to embody.

1. Identify Your Boundary Role Model

Think of someone you know who you admire, or even a public figure who naturally embodies the boundary or air of self-assuredness you aspire to. This could be someone who sets clear limits, maintains their energy, or is unapologetic about protecting their time.

2. Visualize Your Boundary

Imagine this person in a scenario where they're embodying this boundary. Pay attention to their posture, words, and expressions, and to how they engage with others. Notice how they're able to maintain their space without overexplaining or seeking approval. Bring your awareness to the energy and confidence this person projects. Imagine this quality being available to you. Picture yourself embodying the same calm strength and enforcing boundaries that are firm but compassionate. How will you be embodying this boundary going forward? How will your posture, voice, or way of being change?

3. Embodiment Activation

With one hand on your heart, take a deep, cleansing breath and affirm this embodiment activation as a promise to yourself that you will protect your energy. Repeat this whenever you need to strengthen your connection with your new boundary.

> *I honor my energy and protect my peace. I embody boundaries that serve my growth, and I feel grounded, clear, and empowered within them. With each breath, I express this strength, trusting that my boundaries align with my well-being and attract people and experiences that respect my space.*

4. Embodiment in Action

Your final step is to embody your new boundary in a real-life situation. My guess is that you won't need to wait too long for the opportunity to do this, as the Universe has a way of helping us grow and evolve just when we need it. With practice, your new boundaries will become an authentic part of who you are. It's natural to feel a little uncomfortable with change at first, so remember to breathe deeply and feel a sense of groundedness to the Earth as you practice embodying boundaries. You may want to journal about any shifts you observe in interactions or how you feel about your boundaries, noticing any areas where you feel more balanced, protected, or respected.

Speak Your Boundaries

While embodying your boundaries is powerful, at times you may also feel the need to speak your boundaries. This can be uncomfortable, especially at first, but it's helpful to remember that speaking your boundaries isn't about controlling others, but rather about taking responsibility for your emotional, physical, and energetic well-being. Using I statements, such as "I need," or "I feel," makes boundary-setting feel less accusatory and more about your personal experience, which can encourage others to respond supportively. Speaking your boundaries is also about consistency—maintaining and reinforcing them over time shows others that you take your needs seriously. You can maintain strong embodied and spoken boundaries with warmth and kindness, without overexplaining or apologizing—doing this can be a bit of an art form. Having to repeat boundaries may feel robotic at times, especially if we aim to deliver them in a kind way. Instead of feeling awkward or caving in to repeated requests, try to accept the fact that repeating our boundaries is just part of the process, and that the need for it should diminish over time as we embody them more fully. Let's review some tips for speaking our boundaries.

- Practice taking time to assess requests instead of immediately agreeing, and craft polite phrases that help you give yourself more time to decide, such as "Thanks for inviting me. I will need to check my schedule because I may have another commitment on that day, but I'll get back to you tomorrow to let you know."

- Create some go-to phrases for when you do need to decline invitations and requests. Here's an example: "That sounds like a wonderful opportunity, but at the moment I have a family commitment that takes priority and I need to give my full attention to."

- Expressing gratitude by showing appreciation before stating your boundary can set a positive tone. You might say "I really appreciate your understanding" before expressing your need for time or space.

- Practice using sentences starting with *I* rather than *you* to keep the conversation centered on your needs instead of sounding like you're blaming the other person. For example, you could say "I need some alone time to recharge" or "I'm feeling stretched by additional responsibilities at the moment."

- Boundaries aren't about who's right and who's wrong. In most situations, both parties genuinely believe they're doing the right thing or, at the very least, the best they can. Protecting your energy doesn't mean the other person is wrong; it's simply an act of self-care for your own well-being and an opportunity to create space for mutual respect.

- Before communicating a boundary with a loved one, take a moment to visualize your message being well received and acknowledged. Feel the relief of gaining mutual understanding. Lower your shoulders; breathe deeply. Release anxiety with each exhalation.

- Sometimes we need to assert ourselves in a stronger way. When this occurs, speak in direct language without apologizing. Allow your decisive tone to convey the message that you're not available for the situation or conversation. You may want to take a break by physically leaving the room.

The Surrendered Brain

During the luteal phase, the brain naturally shifts gears, creating the perfect space for deeper self-reflection, emotional processing, and aligning with what truly matters. The hormonal interplay of rising progesterone and declining estrogen significantly impacts brain function and mood. Progesterone interacts with the prefrontal cortex, promoting deep thought and emotional processing.[1] The natural shift toward introspection helps us process emotions more fully and build a stronger connection between feelings and intentions. Progesterone also influences the default mode network, a brain system that's active during rest, daydreaming, and introspection.[2] This enhances self-reflective thinking and allows subconscious thoughts and emotions to surface, making this an opportune time for inner work—fostering clarity about our emotions, personal values, and long-term goals. We may crave more downtime as progesterone instills calming and sedative effects on the brain and body. This is due to its interaction with gamma-aminobutyric acid (GABA) receptors in the brain. GABA is a neurotransmitter that supports sleep and promotes relaxation and recovery and reduces stress.[3] Meanwhile, as the estrogen level drops, the brain experiences reduced serotonin and dopamine activity, which can result in heightened emotional sensitivity, lower energy, and a need for more intentional effort to stay motivated.[4] This decline can explain the shifts in mood, increased irritability, and heightened self-criticism, but it also encourages slowing down, appreciating progress, and making a more authentic alignment with personal priorities. Fluctuations in hormone levels can also enhance activity in areas like the amygdala (which processes emotional responses) and the sensory cortex (which is responsible for processing sensory input). This intensified neural activity can lead to a heightened awareness of the surroundings, including increased sensitivity to sounds, smells, and touch. Our increased sensitivity, both internal and external, at this time creates the groundwork for deep emotional processing, problem-solving, and greater self-awareness. It also amplifies our intuition and ability to perceive nuances, fostering clarity about what aligns with our true desires and what may need to be released.

Surrender Phase Practices

Like a treasure chest of precious gems, here is your vault of inner-work practices to help you create the kind of quantum inner shifts that can't help but be reflected in your reality. Each time you cycle around to the Surrender phase, you may want to get cozy, light a candle, and choose one or two of these practices to delve into.

Let Go of How

At this stage of the cycle, you may already notice signs of your desired manifestations' fulfillment, or feel as though they are just around the corner! This is a great frequency to hold—one of positive expectation. Often, our minds will gravitate toward figuring out *how* our manifestations might arrive for us, and this kind of thinking might not be conducive to receiving what we want. Our brains like to solve problems, which becomes burdensome because it can bring our attention to limitations. A better approach would be to hold on to your sense of positive expectation for as long as possible, and to keep returning to it when your mind tries stubbornly to figure out the *how*. To help with this, you can take small actions to open your mind to the myriad of possibilities that the Universe has to offer. This exercise is about creating pathways to help activate several possibilities for good things to flow your way without attaching to any singular outcome. As you practice this, you'll start to see how many avenues there are to invite abundance into your life. The goal is to enjoy the process, knowing you're opening channels for potential opportunities with minimal effort while cultivating a sense of positive anticipation and expectation. Anything can happen!

Exercise:

Choose three or more actions to take from the list below, or come up with your own to try:

- Buy a lottery or raffle ticket.
- Join wait lists for free tickets to museum exhibits, community activities, workshops and trainings, beta

- product tests, wellness classes, or in-demand volunteer roles at special events.
- If you have an entrepreneurial idea, share it with a few trusted friends. Let them know what kind of support would help you bring it to life, and ask them to keep an eye out for people or opportunities that could assist in making it happen.
- Share a gift wish list with friends and family.
- Post on social platforms about something you want to learn, achieve, or acquire. Friends or acquaintances might unexpectedly help, or know someone who can.
- If you offer a product or service, post it on a site and ask for your dream fee.
- If you're looking for love, tell some trusted friends that you are open to meeting potential dates, and consider joining a reputable dating app or service or attending singles events.
- Research small business grants, creative contests, or awards in your field and apply—even if you think the chances are slim.
- Consider investing a small amount (that you're okay letting go of) in a stock or asset you believe could increase in value. Do some research and go with a brand or organization you feel good about.
- Send a pitch or proposal to a potential client, collaborator, or publisher, outlining a clear, compelling idea. One yes opens at least one door, and maybe more.

- Enter competitions to win prizes, trips, or experiences that light you up.

- Boost visibility for your talent. Write a blog, film a video, or start a podcast about an area of interest to attract like-minded individuals.

- Try traveling by a different route, exploring a new café, or attending a random event to invite in unexpected encounters and embrace the power of possibility.

- Create an artwork, song, or downloadable digital item (such as a template, checklist, ebook or guide) based on your unique talent, knowledge, or experience to sell online.

- Engage in online forums or communities and participate in conversations related to your goals or interests. Connections often lead to opportunities.

- As a symbolic act of abundance, declutter an area of your home, and while you are clearing it out, imagine that you're creating space for new blessings to flow in.

- Launch a small crowdfunding campaign for a project you're passionate about. Even small contributions can build momentum.

- Put an item that you no longer want on an auction site to sell to the highest bidder.

By embracing small actions to open up new possibilities, you break through resistance and strengthen your positive expectation that good things can flow your way!

Finding Magic in the Mess

Frustration, complaints, a critical eye, and heightened emotional sensitivity may surface during the Surrender phase and have the potential to clutter your state of mindfulness. Instead of feeling discouraged, harness these natural tendencies as powerful tools to spark *new* desires and fuel your manifestations.

Whether it's the duality of the quarter moon or the grounding, no-nonsense influence of your hormones at play, you may experience a heightened sense of clarity at this time, helping you see through illusions and clear out anything that doesn't serve you. This is a period of discernment, allowing for a resolution for what's been lacking. Although it's an increasingly restful time, it can be quite productive if you listen to your inner guidance and take small actions to elevate your reality. The perspective of this inner guidance is tinted with a critical lens—it may feel as though you are channeling your inner editor in chief as you decisively revise and refine your life. The Surrender phase prompts a natural desire for order and completion, making it a powerful period for refinement and intentional change. This can help you bring projects to completion, tie loose ends, tidy up, clear out, and streamline, fiercely decluttering anything outdated and making swift decisions to eliminate and transmute the old into the new.

When I find myself deep in the energies of the Surrender phase (especially under the gaze of a quarter moon), I begin to notice things that irritate me—in particular anything that doesn't flow around the home. I'm a girl who loves a seamless, connected home, one that has a voice-activated device to dim the lights and play "electronic chill" music as mocktail hour approaches. Electrical outlets are plentiful, and my bathroom alone requires several additional socket extensions because there is always a facial, dental, or hairstyling device being charged. Although I have a lot of love for my many electrical companions, I can't ignore my distaste for the unsightly adaptors and cords that can accumulate. My calm-and-collected nature is put into a spin whenever I have to contend with interwoven masses of cords and chargers. Then there's the wonky outlet extender in the kitchen that never seems to work, the thermostat that periodically shows a low-battery warning, and the air purifier with the blinking light signaling it's time to replace the filter. Why can't technology just work seamlessly in the background of our lives like it's supposed to? Surveying my home with a steely glare, I become hyperaware of anything that doesn't flow. Anything that needs to be upgraded, upcycled, rejected, corrected, or edited becomes obvious. Once identified, I swiftly solve the problem with just a few clicks. Whether it's ordering fresh batteries, researching charging hubs, or subscribing to regular deliveries of items I'm running low on, by investing a few moments to find solutions to my frustrations, I've upgraded my life for months or years to come—creating less stress and more physical and mental clarity.

There are things that can be resolved rather quickly, like my digital dilemmas, and then there are things that might require deeper exploration to extract the magic from the mess. Frustration can be a powerful sign that you're ready for change. Instead of viewing it as negative, harness your critical eye to identify areas for growth or improvement. Let it push you to think creatively and find innovative solutions to challenges. By viewing frustration as a cue for growth, you can transmute lack into desire and resolution.

Exercise:

In your journal, follow the MAGIC formula whenever an irritation pops up:

MESS: State the issue that's irritating you.

ASSESS: Allow yourself to vent and express the disturbance you feel in detail.

GOOD-FEELING DESIRES: What new desires are born out of this frustration?

IDEAS: Brainstorm some ways in which your new desires could become manifested.

CLARITY: What next step will you move forward with?

Example:

MESS: I never know what to prepare for lunch, and there's so little time in the morning that I just grab quick, unhealthy, and expensive snacks and drinks on the go. I need to stop this!

ASSESS: This makes me feel disorganized, rushed, and stressed, and then I get tired after eating unhealthy foods and drinks. I feel like there's never enough time, and when I buy healthy ingredients I feel too tired to chop and prepare them during the week, so they often go to waste. I'm trying to grow my career and spend quality time with family and friends. This lunch situation is adding pressure.

GOOD-FEELING DESIRES: I wish I had a personal chef or someone to drop off lunches for me each day, and I'd also like to cook some meals myself, but only on Sundays. I'd like to have a system to get myself organized without adding more tasks and stress to my plate.

IDEAS: Start meal prep on Sundays. Research a delivery service for fresh, healthy meals. Research a system to organize my recipes and an online grocery list that I can access on my tablet and phone and add items to using a voice recognition device while

I'm in the kitchen. Ask family members to help with meal prep to lighten my load.

CLARITY: I'm going to stick a calendar on the fridge and plan my lunches ahead of time, starting this weekend. I'll have fun with it and play music while I prep. I'll also research meal-delivery options for busy weeks when I have a lot of projects and events happening.

Now it's your turn!

MESS:

ASSESS:

GOOD-FEELING DESIRES:

IDEAS:

CLARITY:

When you resolve everyday issues that need improvement, you're up-leveling your lifestyle *now* instead of waiting for something big to change in the future. By making small enhancements during each Surrender phase, over time you can elevate your life in a way that compounds and supports you beautifully.

Somatic Moment: Tension Release Ritual

Have you ever caught yourself hunched over, jaw clenched, or holding your breath while lost in stressful thoughts or tasks? Stress often causes a disconnect between the mind and body. In these moments, somatic practices can help you to reengage with your body to release tension, process emotions, and regulate your nervous system, bringing you back into harmony.

By pausing to take a few deep breaths, adjusting your posture, and gently shaking out tension from your shoulders and arms, you can create an immediate and powerful shift. These simple somatic practices train you to recognize tension as it arises and transition from a stressed state to a calmer, more grounded one. Over time, these shifts invite greater ease, spaciousness, and creativity, helping you approach challenges with renewed energy and focus.

Somatic practices emphasize the mind-body connection, using physical sensations, intentional movement, self-massage, body-centered meditation, and breath work to support balance and well-being.

Exercise:

1. Find a comfortable seated position, then close your eyes and take a few deep, calming breaths to center yourself.

2. Tune in to the sensation of tension in your body. Where do you feel it? Visualize this tension as a cloud and give it a color.

3. Continue to breathe deeply, and with each exhalation, visualize the cloud of tension leaving your body with your breath. Imagine your tension dissolving into the air and drifting away.

4. Gently press on your forehead with your fingertips. Massage in circular motions, focusing on the space between your eyebrows. This helps signal your body to relax and reduce mental clutter.

5. Finish by focusing on your body's calm response. Feel the sensation of relaxation spreading from your forehead down to your toes. Take a moment to note how this feels.

Consider integrating this Tension Release Ritual into your regular routine, especially during the Surrender phase. This can help build resilience to stress and support deeper self-awareness.

Allowing Natural Consequences

As women, we're often juggling so much. Imagine being able to trust and let go a little. But what would happen if we allowed others to step in, take ownership, and share their strengths?

Coaching client Lila was experiencing anxiety, weight gain, fatigue, digestive issues, and other unwanted symptoms due to a hormonal imbalance. She was seeking support in implementing a few lifestyle shifts to complement her treatments for thyroid dysfunction, so we reviewed her stress level. It became clear that as a newlywed who was settling into a brand-new home, spending time with an ailing parent, and bearing responsibility for the launch of a new work project, Lila was being pulled in many directions and feeling overwhelmed. She hadn't had time to focus on her own well-being, not to mention pause for a bit of fun now and then. Something had to give. When we looked at what she could let go of, at first she didn't feel like there was anything to relinquish or anyone who could help her out, yet the tasks she was taking on appeared to intersect with the responsibilities of others. She also recounted a few common stressful scenarios, like her new husband leaving unwashed dishes on the kitchen counter, her siblings being too busy to visit their parent, and her co-worker always needing help with last-minute tasks. "What would happen if you just stopped taking on the burden of these stressful things?" I asked.

Sometimes it feels as though the Earth would spin off its axis if we even attempted to channel a portion of our time and energy into our own wellness, beauty, pleasure, curiosity, creativity, or dreams. But have we ever really tested this theory? What if we politely declined taking on additional burdens and responsibilities and just allowed natural consequences to unfold? Things might get messy—at least for a while, but then... perhaps they'd get better. Much better. By employing an unbothered "natural consequences" approach to certain stressors that don't belong to us, we get to conserve our energy, remove ourselves from the discomfort of verbal conflict, and accept the notion that other adults are competent individuals.

At first, we may feel guilty when we practice conserving energy, but I'll let you in on a little secret: Men do it all the time! Before you blow a fuse, you should know that they're probably not even aware they are doing this—it's kind of hardwired. From an evolutionary perspective, men's bodies seem to balance energy use to support bursts of testosterone-driven activity, like hunting or protecting resources. Their metabolism appears to conserve energy during less demanding periods, helping maintain stamina and efficiency for tasks requiring sudden, intensive exertion.[5] Historically, men's roles demanded repeated bouts of physical activity, which helped shape these metabolic adaptations. In today's world, this might show up as him saying he'll do something but waiting awhile to see if someone else will do it first. Oftentimes a competent, resourceful woman will jump in to save the day. Sound familiar? When couples get into this pattern, it can unintentionally result in the man feeling useless, criticized, or unappreciated, and the woman feeling overburdened, resentful, or like the parent in the relationship. The romantic polarity and playfulness are then in danger of waning.

So instead of jumping in to take on more or playing the waiting game, stop the clock and enjoy a half day at the spa, bookstore, or hiking trail—whatever you need to do to be unavailable to rescue other people from their tasks. We're not talking about just letting *everything* slide, only the things that aren't truly yours to begin with. Helping and supporting others is part of being in a relationship, whether it's romantic partners, friends, family members, or co-workers, but you are not required to constantly fix things or take on other people's responsibilities to the detriment of your own well-being. By protecting your energy you can share from your overflow, not from a place of stress or lack.

As for Lila, after a few days of kitchen messiness her husband stepped up to take charge of loading and unloading the dishwasher each day. When she wasn't available to drive across town to pick up her siblings to visit their parent, they ordered a ride, and when she chose to spend a relaxing evening at home with her husband instead of staying late to rescue her disorganized co-worker, the assignment was completed with the help of an intern who appreciated the challenge.

Your task, should you choose to accept it, is to be mindful of opportunities for allowing natural consequences to unfold during this Surrender phase. Yes, it's going to be uncomfortable at first, but soon you'll be gracefully sidestepping unnecessary burdens with a twinkle in your eye and a *lot* more energy to expend on propelling *your* dreams into motion.

Exercise:

Choose three or more of these journal prompts to explore the practice of allowing natural consequences to unfold.

- Have you taken responsibility for something that isn't truly yours to manage? How can you allow others to step into their own responsibility?

- What fears arise when you consider stepping back and allowing things to unfold on their own? How might you soothe those fears without taking action?

- How do you practice patience in situations where results take time? What helps you stay grounded while waiting?

- If you released control over a certain situation in your life, how might that create more freedom, energy, or peace for you?

- When have you experienced flow or ease by not overplanning or controlling? What allowed you to stay flexible, and how did it change the outcome?

- Think of a recent situation in which you didn't intervene. What natural consequences unfolded? What did you learn from watching rather than acting?

- Think about a project that feels overwhelming. In what ways could you step back from the stressful parts? What would happen if you let go of perfection or delegated some of the work?

- Write about a time when stepping back led to a better outcome than expected. How can you apply that experience to a current challenge?

- How would it feel to let go of the need to ensure a specific outcome? What could you gain from enjoying the process?

- Where are you spending energy in trying to control situations? Could that energy be better spent on activities that bring you joy or fulfillment?

- What feelings arise when you don't jump in to resolve an issue immediately? How can you sit with those feelings instead of acting on them?

Conserve Energy by Honoring Your Ultradian Rhythms

As you learned in Chapter 2, the monthly cycle you're aligning with now (either menstrual or moon) is called an infradian rhythm. Your daily sleep-wake cycle is regulated by the 24-hour circadian rhythm, but you also cycle through ultradian rhythms that are approximately 90 to 120 minutes long. The body's energy and attention are optimal as the rhythm peaks before needing a break.[6] Monitor yourself for the subtle cues of your body—such as restlessness, hunger, thirst, fatigue, fidgeting, and nervous tension—and try to honor her need for short periods of rest throughout the day. Taking these breaks allows for mind-body regulation, when our minds and bodies have an opportunity to sort through incoming data. As we move through the day, our body is processing metabolic waste and other by-products of our productivity. Breaks give our cells a chance to perform important repair work, and help our immune system respond effectively to challenges.

But instead of honoring these signals, we often push harder, ignoring cravings, skipping rest, and engaging in high-intensity activities. Over time, this stress can lead to dysregulation—disrupted cortisol levels, sleep cycles, and even metabolism—causing inflammation, trouble sleeping, fatigue, burnout, and more serious health challenges. Hustle culture and the "no days off" approach to success encourage relentless productivity and unbroken streaks of daily habit completion, yet this ideal clashes with the natural rhythms of a woman's hormonal cycle. Our body's intricate balance of hormones is highly sensitive to stress and overexertion, making this kind of approach counterproductive to long-term health.

During the luteal phase, when the progesterone level rises and estrogen declines, we often experience increased cravings, a desire for comfort, and a greater need for rest and nourishment. These are signals that your body is engaging in vital processes, such as thickening the uterine lining (the endometrium) and managing the hormonal dance that supports overall health. This behind-the-scenes effort requires more calories, less physical exertion, and extra self-care.

Fueling ourselves with nutrient-dense foods and adequate rest during the luteal phase can enhance our physical and emotional well-being. Cravings for warmth and comfort reflect our body's need for grounding and nurturing energy. Gentle restorative practices like yoga and walking can feel more supportive than intense workouts. Embrace self-compassion and understand that productivity looks different in each phase. Honoring your cycle, and your need for rest, doesn't mean stepping away from ambition—it means working smarter, not harder, in alignment with your body's innate wisdom.

Choosing habits that fit into 15- to 20-minute blocks during your daytime schedule offers your mind and body much-needed breaks. Aligning with ultradian rhythms not only conserves energy, but also promotes greater emotional and physical wellness. By integrating intuitive movement, reflective practices, fresh air, screen-free breaks, and balanced nourishment, you can optimize focus, sustain energy, and enhance well-being throughout the day.

Let's review some top tips for ultradian rhythm breaks:

- Try practices that relieve stress and reset energy, such as breathing exercises or intentionally releasing unwanted thoughts, worries, and stresses. This reduces emotional strain and promotes a balanced, mindful approach to productivity.

- Eat nourishing meals and snacks aligned with your natural hunger cues to support metabolic health, energy regulation, cognitive function, and a steady mood.

- Choose light movement that matches your energy level. Walking or stretching do wonders to circulate blood and release stress without overexertion. This allows the body to stay engaged without taxing your energy supply.

- In the afternoon, when your energy dips, perform gentler activities to honor the natural rhythm, enhancing cortisol balance and preventing adrenal fatigue

- Engage in a screen-free hobby or craft. This helps the brain clear mental clutter and boosts creativity and clarity.

- Spending time outdoors exposes you to natural light, which supports your circadian rhythms and boosts mood-enhancing hormones. Fresh air and movement also reduce stress and increase mental clarity, helping you feel more grounded and refreshed.

Exercise:

Write down a few ideas for activities you'd enjoy doing during your ultradian rhythm breaks of 15 to 20 minutes. Consider when you can intentionally take these breaks throughout your day (ideally about every 90 to 120 minutes) and incorporate them into your schedule.

Detach to Attract

Now is the perfect time to help your manifestations be activated into fruition by gently releasing your attachment to them. It may strike you as counterintuitive at first, but it's all about shifting from a mindset of scarcity and control to one of abundance and trust.

Let's take a look at scarcity. Desiring something you don't yet have to the point of obsessing over it, worrying about it, or not being able to feel happy without it is giving the energy of lack. There's a tendency to glorify our desires before they manifest, but have you ever noticed that after receiving them, they rarely turn out to be as perfect as you imagined they would be? While our desired manifestations can bring us significant joy, they won't be long-term cure-alls for the complexities of life. They might enhance our lives, but challenges will persist, and new desires will continue to emerge. Recognizing this gives us perspective, and a healthy level of detachment so that we can be open to all opportunities instead of being fixated on one particular outcome.

When it comes to the topic of control, by releasing our tight grip on how things *should* be, we allow the natural unfolding of our path, inviting synchronicities and unexpected opportunities. This approach transforms desire from a force that consumes to a creative force that guides, helping us navigate life's twists and turns with grace and resilience. By cultivating a state of flow, you can learn to trust that the Universe has a plan far greater than your own singular vision. You open yourself up to the possibility of a partnership with the Divine, allowing it to bring forth manifestations in ways you might never have considered. The concept of trusting the Universe (or Source, or Creation) doesn't have to feel far-fetched. Think about the structure, stability, and support available in the breath, the sunrise and sunset, and the ever-flowing cycles of days and seasons.

Exercise:

To help cultivate healthy detachment and a sense of surrender and openness to blessings, think about what it is you want to manifest and reflect on three or more of these questions:

- Q: What if the outcome I'm hoping for isn't exactly what I expect or need? Can I imagine other ways for my desires to manifest or be fulfilled?

- Q: Is my desired manifestation a *need* or a *want*? What is it that I really need?

- Q: How do I want my desired manifestation to make me feel? Are there things already in my life that make me feel this way?

- Q: In what ways am I glorifying the thing I want to manifest? How might I still feel complete and happy even if I don't get it?

- Q: What might I learn or how might I grow from letting go of this attachment? How could releasing this desire open up space for something even better?

- Q: How does holding on to this desire impact my present moment? Am I creating stress, anxiety, or a sense of lack?

- Q: Am I willing to trust the process and let go of the need to control the outcome? How can I bring more faith and ease into my approach to manifesting?

- Q: In what ways am I already trusting the Universe? How could I expand on the feeling of support that gives me?

- Q: What has the journey of manifesting taught me? What am I discovering along the way?

By releasing control and attachment, you cultivate trust and allow the Universe to bring what is best for you in unexpected ways. Surrender to the reality that your heart and soul desires are already a part of you. There is no lack.

Evidence of Alignment

While patiently awaiting your desired manifestation to take shape, you may notice hints of it appearing in your environment. Maybe you hear a stranger mention a goal similar to yours or you spot visual symbols that remind you of what you've been calling in. Rather than feeling left out when you see your desires reflected in other people's lives, take it as a positive signal that your desired manifestation is aligning with your energy. This phenomenon ties into the brain's reticular activating system (RAS), a network that filters information and highlights what's relevant to you. When you set an intent on or a goal—whether it's manifesting a dream job, a relationship, or a lifestyle goal—the RAS begins filtering your environment to highlight signs, opportunities, or patterns connected to it.[7] This is why, once you focus on something, you might feel like it's popping up everywhere. It's not just about coincidence; your brain is actively recognizing patterns and connections that support your vision. Every symbol, mention, or moment of synchronicity is a reminder of what's possible. Celebrate these hints as evidence that what you desire is aligning with your reality. The RAS responds to visuals, so make time to look at pictures or visual representations of your desires and imagine the feelings they will bring you.

Trigger Workshop

A colleague takes credit for your idea during a meeting. Your partner forgets your anniversary. A friend shuts down in mid-conversation and walks away. Throughout life we're tested with challenging situations, and it can be all-too-easy to carry unhealed emotions along for the ride. Since the Surrender phase is conducive to releasing and letting go, this can be an opportune time to alchemize the emotional reactions that arise when you feel triggered. Triggers often point to unresolved emotions, unmet needs, or hidden opportunities for growth. We can harness these moments as powerful tools for self-awareness, healing, and alignment with our true desires. In this workshop, we'll turn those unsettling moments into drivers for meaningful change, release emotional baggage, and become empowered with new insights to take forward in our lives.

When I thought about it, I realized that this exercise was the catalyst for this entire book. I'd created a few self-reflection steps to guide myself through triggering situations that used to overwhelm me with emotion and lead to anxiety. I found the steps helpful, so I shared them with friends and clients, who also found them helpful. I had initially planned to publish a guided journal so that other people could also work through these steps and be able to transform activated emotions into something that served them, but as the idea of the journal evolved and took on momentum, I began incorporating additional inner-work tools, and the project gradually transformed into this book.

This exercise is designed to address mild emotional triggers, not deeply upsetting or traumatic experiences. On a scale of 1 to 10, we'll focus on situations that feel like a 3 or lower in intensity (everyone's nervous system processes situations differently, so your 3 might be someone else's 8, and vice versa). Like all exercises in this book, it's completely optional, so feel free to skip it or revisit it later when it feels right for you. Are you ready to release stuck energy and lighten your load?

Exercise:

There's something therapeutic about getting your thoughts out of your mind and onto paper so you can observe them from a different vantage point. Grab your journal and follow the prompts.

Trigger: A situation sparked an emotional response.

1. Name the feeling: What feeling or feelings were activated by this situation?

2. Your response: What did you feel in your body? How did you react externally?

3. Recall the past: Has this same feeling, or mixture of feelings, come up in the past? What's your earliest memory of feeling this way?

4. Find meaning: If there is a lesson tied to this situation, what could that be? Is there something that needs to be healed? Is it revealing a limiting belief or an old story you may need to release?

5. Re-create: If you could go back in time and adjust your response to the situation, would you do anything differently?

6. Elevate: Imagine a future version of yourself, not too far from now, living a life where your heart and soul desires have been fulfilled. You feel truly content and are able to effortlessly bring your dreams into reality. If a similar triggering situation comes up again, how would this future version of you handle it?

7. Release: If there is an emotion, regret, or response tied to this situation that needs to be released, what would that be?

Example:

Trigger: A colleague took credit for my idea in a meeting.

1. Name the feeling: shocked, betrayed, insignificant, angry

2. Your response: I felt frozen in the moment and didn't say anything. I felt shut down during the rest of the meeting and couldn't concentrate properly.

3. Recall the past: I felt this way in the past when one of my parents would overrule my requests and disregard my feelings.

4. Find meaning: I find it difficult to be assertive and speak up for myself. I notice that it's much easier for other people to do that. I'd like to try voicing my opinion more often going forward. I commit to respecting myself in this way from now on.

5. Re-create: I would have gathered the courage to politely confront my colleague after the meeting to ask why she took credit for my idea.

6. Elevate: My more confident future self would smile and make a cute remark in the meeting about how she must have forgotten that it was my idea.

7. Release: I forgive myself for not speaking up and voicing my concern with my colleague. I release my anger around this situation and take the lesson as a gift.

Now it's your turn!

Well done for facing your emotional triggers head-on—it's definitely easier said than done, but having worked through them, don't you feel much lighter, more empowered, and wiser? You may find it helpful to follow this exercise with a releasing technique from the next section.

Releasing Techniques

When you no longer wish to feel weighed down by difficult emotions, limiting beliefs, critical self-talk, or burdens from the past and you're ready to surrender to a lighter way of being, try one or more of these releasing techniques to help elevate your energetic point of attraction.

Fire Ritual

Write down on a piece of paper whatever it is you'd like to release. Use a fireproof plate or vessel and go outside and burn the paper. Flames are a visual representation of transformation. Visualize the emotion being transmuted by Source energy into pure, golden light. Alternatively, light a candle while focusing on your intention to release old energy and welcome in new energies.

Inner Child Emotional Release

Begin by gathering some colored pencils, markers, or paints and a blank sheet of paper. Settle into a quiet, comfortable space where you won't be disturbed. Close your eyes and take several deep breaths to center yourself, releasing any tension with each exhalation. Once you feel relaxed, imagine yourself in a safe, serene place—perhaps a cozy room filled with sunlight or a beautiful, peaceful garden. In this space, invite your inner child to join you. Notice their age, emotions, and energy. Allow yourself to connect with compassion and curiosity. Gently begin a dialogue with your inner child, asking them what they need from you, whether it's comfort, understanding, or validation. Listen with openness, honoring their feelings. Reassure them that they are safe and deeply loved, and that they no longer need to carry the burdens of the past. Let them know you're thankful for the ways they've helped you over the years. Affirm to them that as your adult self, you are now capable of handling life's challenges with resiliency, calm, and maturity. Acknowledge their fears and remind them that moving forward, you'll respond to difficult situations with greater inner stability and compassion. Following your conversation, visualize wrapping your inner child in a warm embrace and sharing a sense of unconditional love and acceptance. Imagine any heavy emotions from the past beginning to dissolve. Assign each unwanted emotion a color, and use pencils, markers or paints to release that color onto the paper. As you draw or paint, imagine the emotion flowing out of you and onto the paper, symbolically releasing it from your body. When you feel the process is complete, discard or destroy the paper to release old burdens and create space for new, supportive energy.

Share Your Story

Sharing your story with a trusted friend or family member or a professional therapist or healer can be profoundly healing. When someone who's supportive witnesses and validates your feelings, it can relieve you of the burden of carrying those emotions alone. I don't believe we're meant to live in shame and regret for years. By shining light on our shadows, we can dissolve their hold on us and release the weight of dense emotions, unlocking our full potential to manifest our dreams.

Sacred Space

Visualize a magical place where you feel completely safe. That place may be your inner temple. Take a moment to imagine your glorious, harmonious, relaxing, and comforting space. Design it in your imagination. Create a place where you can sit comfortably, and adjust the temperature so it's perfect for what you are craving. Request that Source energy imbue your sacred space with healing light. Imagine entering your sacred space to relax and dwell there in a beautiful healing light. Rest and release any emotions that need to be cleared as your energy body is being restored and cleansed. Return to your sacred space as often as you like to rejuvenate yourself on an energetic level.

Dancing Through Emotion

When emotions feel overwhelming, our bodies often carry the weight of that energy. Movement, especially dance, can be a powerful tool for releasing pent-up feelings and reconnecting with a sense of freedom and flow. Dancing through emotion begins with somatic practices for nervous system regulation and then gives way to expressive movement and dance with the intention of releasing emotional energies from the body, mind, and spirit. Find a quiet, private space where you feel comfortable moving freely. Begin by choosing music that feels soothing or uplifting. Take some deep breaths to get grounded and connect to your body. Once you've tuned in to your body, start engaging in small, slow movements that invite release, like shaking out the arms, gently rolling the neck, or swaying the torso. As your nervous system starts to settle, you can begin transitioning into freer, more fluid movements that encourage self-expression. Move in a way that feels intuitive, allowing your body to speak, tapping in to unconscious emotions and bringing them to the surface. As you dance, breathe deeply and with each exhale release the energy you no longer need. You might even visualize the emotion leaving your body like a mist dissolving into the air. Finish by gently brushing your arms and legs in downward movements with your hands, imagining that you are sweeping old energies out of your body. Take a moment to stand still, close your eyes, and place your hands over your heart. Thank yourself for showing up and releasing what no longer serves you.

A Lifestyle Surrendered

Align your lifestyle with the Surrender phase, whether it's within your personal cycle or that of the new moon. Here are some ideas you may wish to explore:

Mind:

- Review your projects and tie up any loose ends. Finalize what needs to be completed.

- Embrace comfort wherever you can and begin to rest and restore yourself in preparation for a new cycle.

- Embrace any emotional-release urges that come to the surface. Watch a movie or show that allows you to feel a range of emotions or to release emotions through tears.

- Pursue hobbies and crafts projects that help you feel creative or lift your mood to embrace a sense of calmness.

- Explore mindfulness practices like breath work, meditation, or yoga nidra to soothe heightened emotions and develop mental clarity.

- Use a critical eye to see things that need improving, and keep a notebook or notes app handy to write them down. If you sense a big new idea or desire bubbling up, make a note to revisit it during the next Attune phase.
- Diffuse essential oils with relaxing qualities, such as lavender or rose.

Body:

- Embrace ease and flow by cutting back on stimulants where possible. Consider taking a break from caffeine, or at least decreasing your consumption.
- Relax your nervous system with somatic practices like connecting with your five senses. Touch your arms gently, tune in to sounds around you, notice something you see that's interesting, identify scents in the air and take one slow, deep breath in and out through your mouth, feeling yourself become centered, calm, and fully present.
- Feed your adrenal glands by grazing on fruits and vegetables and consuming natural herbal teas. Consider supplements with calming or adaptogenic effects such as magnesium or ashwagandha.
- Enjoy slow-burning complex carbs and high-fiber foods like root vegetables, lentils, and oats. Snack on foods that reduce bloating and are liver-friendly such as herbal teas and low-fat, plant-rich meals.
- Hydrate your body with lots of fluids, such as coconut water, that contain natural electrolytes.

- Choose comfortable clothing that is not restrictive and allows you to move freely.

- Indulge in a massage, steam room, or sauna session; body brushing; or gentle exfoliation to relieve tension.

- For maximum growth, wait until the next waxing moon to trim your hair.

- Choose exercises that help you release tension at an intensity that feels right. Light stretching, Pilates, yoga, and other low-intensity workouts will help you avoid spikes in cortisol.

Soul:

- Spend quality time with loved ones and create meaningful moments to enhance your mood and boost your feel-good hormones.

- Journal to release your thoughts onto paper.

- Refrain from staring at the moon while she is waning. Save moon watching for when she is waxing or full.

Transitioning to the Next Cycle

Now that you have built trust in yourself, your Divine Downloads, and your ability to live your desires into reality, practice the Attune phase Heart and Soul Desires Meditation on page 63 again with a renewed level of trust in what your heart and soul are telling you. Tune in to see if your desires have changed or remain the same.

Chapter 8

CYCLE MASTERY

Congratulations! You have completed one full cycle. Now it's time to master your art. With each rotation of a cycle you create more and more magnetism and momentum, a phenomenon known as the *compounding effect*. If you didn't have time to do the Cycle Magic exercises during a phase of your cycle and had to skip them, don't worry. But also don't give up—just continue from where you are. The beauty of this system is that you have another opportunity just around the corner to delve into the exercises, and then again after that. Keep turning and returning. It's always here for you. If you are aligning with your menstrual cycle and it gets out of whack for any reason, try gently transitioning to the moon cycle.

The more we can practice being the kind of person who makes their dreams a priority, the more likely we are to manifest them. We learn and retain information best through embodiment, not intellect alone. In this chapter you'll find some more advanced topics and exercises to help you become an unstoppable manifester.

Portals

Now that you're accustomed to working with the energies of cycles and rhythms, you will likely be able to identify other energetic windows that you can leverage, like portals. A portal is an energetic gateway or opening that allows access to another reality or state of being—a symbolic threshold through which transformation or connection to other possibilities or states of consciousness can occur. We can use portals to save time and accelerate our manifestations by amplifying our intentions for who we want to become and what we wish to manifest. We do this by consciously focusing on our desires while we are connected to a portal, whether it's at a specific time or location or not. I must confess—I'm in a portal right now. It's that weird stretch of days between Christmas and New Year when no one seems to know what day it is. I'm leveraging this unique time tunnel of stillness and fluidity as my "intentional portal" to focus on crafting my dream project to completion. Here are a few types of portals that you can harness.

Location Portals

Location portals can serve as powerful tools to align yourself with the future you wish to manifest. By physically placing yourself in spaces that resonate with your aspirations, you create a tangible connection to your dreams. Visit locations like a university you aspire to attend, a sports arena where you envision yourself performing, a neighborhood you'd love to live in, or even a town hall where you see yourself making an impact to help anchor your intentions. The resting places of deceased loved ones or spiritual sages can also be used as portals to connect with their energy and ask for support in your earthly journey.

Celestial Portals

There are powerful moments during the year when the cosmos aligns in such a way that it opens energetic portals for transformation and manifestation. Events like the equinoxes, solstices, and the Lion's Gate (peaking in energy on August 8 each year) serve as gateways where it is believed that the veil between the seen and unseen is thinner, allowing us to tap into greater potential and set intentions.

Rituals

We might think of portals as rare occurrences, but the truth is that we can connect with them every day, or even several times a day if we choose. A ritual is a good example of this. Perhaps you could set aside a few minutes each morning or evening to connect with your intentions. This might include clearing the space with a sound bowl, using crystals to amplify a meditation, writing in a journal, making and drinking herbal tea, or more. Rituals can be personal to you, or practiced as part of a spiritual community or group.

Life Transitions

Significant moments in your life such as birthdays, anniversaries, and milestones of personal growth create natural portals for reflection and transformation. These moments often carry a deeper resonance, offering opportunities to pause, honor where you've come from, and recalibrate for where you're heading. Transitions offer a unique window to align with your intentions, set new goals, and manifest the next phase of your journey.

Holidays

Holiday portals are special moments in time when collective energy and tradition converge, creating a unique opportunity to connect with deeper intentions. Celebrations, holidays, and significant dates offer a chance to tap in to the shared spirit of renewal, helping to amplify personal transformation and manifestation through the collective consciousness, spiritual light, or rituals associated with these dates. You might also like to choose a date of personal significance.

Creative Portals

These are moments or environments that inspire creativity and allow new ideas to flow freely. Creative portals can occur when someone is in a flow state, in nature, observing a moving piece of art, taking a moment to rest, or even participating in collaborative settings where the exchange of ideas ignites new thinking.

Symbolic Portals

Symbolic portals are recognized through signs or synchronicities in our waking life. Angel numbers, such as 11:11, serve as powerful reminders of alignment and presence, drawing our attention to moments of transformation and awakening. These portals evoke a sense of protection, guidance, and support while also connecting us to a collective consciousness of energetic flow.

Sacred Texts

Portals often manifest through ancient wisdom and sacred teachings that offer profound insights into the human experience. These texts and stories serve as gateways to spiritual elevation, guiding those who connect with them toward self-realization, clarity, and deeper connections with the Divine or universal truths.

Elemental Portals

Elemental portals are a powerful way to connect with nature's energies to manifest your desires. Water represents emotional flow and intuition. Working with it might include performing rituals involving cleansing baths, setting intentions with moon-charged water, or meditating by the ocean or a river to wash away old patterns. Air embodies clarity and inspiration. Deep breathing, burning sage or palo santo, or whispering affirmations into the wind invites a connection with fresh energy and ideas. Fire signifies transformation and passion. Lighting candles or writing intentions next to a fire can ignite the energy needed for bold action. Earth symbolizes stability and grounding. Planting seeds or working with gemstones or crystals can help anchor your manifestations into reality. By connecting with these elements or spending time in nature, you open energetic gateways that amplify your intentions and align them with the natural world.

Intentional Portals

You can create your own portal by setting aside a specific time frame—perhaps a few days—during which you eliminate all distractions, notifications, and commitments. This allows you to collapse time and focus on an important phase of your wellness or development, such as studying for a final exam, completing a project, doing a cleanse, building a website or program, decluttering your closet, or writing a book. You could also set up an intentional portal for part of your day, assigning it to a particular task or as an "acting as if" practice where you live out part of your day in the way you'd ultimately like to.

Extend Your Target

Once you've put your energy and focus into manifesting a desire over the course of a cycle or two and you start to feel it coming to fruition, it's time to extend your target. This is about looking just beyond your current manifestation and preparing for what's next, even before it fully materializes. It's about mentally and energetically stepping into the next stage—thinking ahead, planning, and aligning with what's to come. This creates momentum with forward-moving energy, staying aligned with your desires and intentions while slightly expanding your vision. Extending your target is a slight shift in focus, like looking through a telescope into the night sky. As you observe a distant star, adjusting the lens slightly shifts your focus to bring a different star into clearer view—you make a subtle change to see something new or beyond your current focus. Or like navigating a trail while hiking—you're aware of the ground under your feet, but also scanning the path ahead, adjusting your focus just enough to anticipate the terrain beyond you.

Exercise:
Think about the thing you really want to manifest. Once you have it, what are some of the next steps you will need to undertake?

Manifestation: Car
Next steps: Start researching things you will need once the car arrives, like window tinting, a personalized license plate, a windshield sticker giving you access to the HOV lane if the car is an electric vehicle, a transponder for paying road tolls, a car cover, and other items to customize the interior and exterior. Be ready with a plan of action.

Manifestation: Entrepreneurial project
Next steps: Planning how to promote your project once it's completed, or imagining what your next big venture might look like, whether it's exploring a new partnership or diving into an entirely new field that aligns with your passions and growth.

Now it's your turn!

Cycle Wisdom

Having engaged with the inner-work exercises and activities throughout your cycle, you will have come to know yourself in a deeper way. You may have gained clearer insight into what you truly want to manifest and how your unique presence can help bring it to life. These self-reflection journal prompts will help crystallize this growth and elevate your experience.

Exercise:
Choose three or more journal prompts to explore.

- Q: Which phase taught you the most about yourself?
- Q: What types of activities will you be putting more time and attention into moving forward?
- Q: What did you learn about your strengths and talents?
- Q: What stories from the past are you letting go of?
- Q: Why are your desired manifestations important to you?
- Q: In what ways are you already manifesting with ease?
- Q: Write about a time when you felt lit up by something and pursued it even though it didn't make logical sense. What did you gain from that experience?
- Q: What forces of misalignment will you be phasing out or minimizing?
- Q: Have any of your initial desires shifted? How so?
- Q: In what areas might you be making things more difficult than they need to be? How can you simplify?

Your Energetic Blueprint

Tools like astrology, Human Design, the Enneagram, numerology, Gene Keys, the Chinese zodiac, or even feng shui can offer insights into your natural strengths, tendencies, and areas for growth. They can provide clarity on your internal energies and how they interact with external forces in your life. This isn't about fortune-telling—it's about understanding the energies you're inherently working with so you can better guide your own destiny. It's much like referring to a GPS system to navigate through life's twists and turns. These energetic insights can help you recognize patterns in your life, showing you where you can align your actions to achieve more ease and flow.

To get an accurate reading, a provider of any of these services will need the date, time, and place of your birth. If you're unsure of the exact time, the service provider may be able to estimate it for you. Energies surround and reside within us, and they influence every aspect of our being, shaping us on multiple levels, both internally and externally. By knowing your unique energetic blueprint, you can harness the power of your true nature and make empowered choices that guide you toward more aligned opportunities in your personal and professional life.

Do you feel called to explore your energetic blueprint? If so, take time to research some of these energetic systems and explore what types of readings or tools they could offer you. Remember, you are in charge of your destiny, and through your free will, you have the power to choose the tools and energies that can support you in manifesting the life you desire.

Cycle Magic Q&A

I know you have questions! Here's where we explore some of the more nuanced aspects related to the Cycle Magic system and alignment with the various cycles and rhythms.

Q: How do I approach the overlap between phases?

As you may have experienced, the energies of the phases tend to overlap slightly. The moon, as a large celestial body, takes its time gently transitioning through each phase of energy. Similarly, your hormone cycle is a living, dynamic force that can vary from month to month, allowing room for flexibility and intuition. For example, the waxing gibbous moon or anticipation of ovulation may fuel the final moments of the Awaken phase or usher in the culmination of the Thrive phase. In these crossover moments, it all comes down to your intention. How will you harness the energy available to you? Will you focus on completing your Awaken phase experiments with the Cycle Habits Tracker, or dive fully into Conscious Embodiment exercises as part of the Thrive phase?

The energy between phases is fluid and transmutable, giving you control and power. Do what feels right for you at any given time. In astrology, our fate isn't determined by the movement of the planets—we are beings of free will using astrology as a cosmic GPS or energetic weather forecast. Once we understand the energetic influences at play, we can use them to our advantage—flowing with them, adapting, or even overriding them when necessary. You are the master of your destiny, and the energies of each phase are powerful tools to help you achieve your goals and dreams.

Q: What if my menstrual cycle and the moon cycle are in opposite phases?

When you're deep in your luteal (Surrender) phase but the moon is at her first quarter, what to do? With some mindfulness and introspection you can still align with the energies that will support you. Here are some approaches that may help you.

- Tune in and spend a few moments breathing with one hand on your heart and one on your belly. How do you feel? Do you have restless energy? Are you at ease? Are you tired? Is there something you're urging yourself to do? What phase are you more in tune with in this moment? On this day?

- Having noted where you are in your cycle in comparison with the moon's position, what does your intuition tell you about the energies available to you today? What do you feel called to do?

- In general, I have found that my own body's rhythm is much stronger and "closer to home" than the moon's influence. My default system, as someone who is not on hormonal birth control, is alignment with my menstrual cycle. The phases feel more visceral and urgent when your body is the antenna for these energies. If my menstrual cycle is having her irregular moments, whether because I'm traveling in a different time zone or flirting with perimenopause, I release any frustration and gently transition to whatever phase the moon is in, and more importantly what energies I intuitively feel I can tune in to on a particular day or stretch of time.

- Now that you are aware of and playing with natural cycles of energy, you get to feel more supported in life. Try some of these affirmations on for size:

    There is always a supportive system of energy available to me.

    I am in control of my destiny and use natural energies to help me co-create.

    There is a rhythm to the Universe, and I ride her waves with ease and flow.

    I gently shift between energies at any time to fuel my goals.

    I am a dynamic feminine being who is co-creating with the Universe.

    I can access my intuition and desires at any time. I just need to tune in.

    I am worthy of my desires, and the Universe supports me.

    I manifest my desires with ease and flow.

Aligning with your menstrual and/or the moon cycle phases is a whole new language of embodiment, but it's also something innate to the feminine being that can feel healing and familiar once we've moved through a few cycles and become accustomed to the energetic phases. I recommend beginning your journey by choosing one system to follow—either the menstrual or moon cycle—and getting used to working with those energies. Then, when you get a feel for the phases, you can primarily use your menstrual cycle and keep an eye on the moon cycle (and astrology at large), as I do. The moon is powerful—no doubt you've heard about its influence on the tides, and therefore on our bodies since we are composed of mostly water—so it can be hugely influential in our lives. You may want to keep track of whether any eclipses are coming up, or any huge transitions between powerful planets such as Jupiter and Saturn. Choose an astrologer you feel aligned with and check in weekly or monthly on what energetic influences might be coming down the pipeline. In this way, you can prepare for the energetic weather ahead.

Q: What's the best approach if I'm in perimenopause?

During this time your hormones can fluctuate wildly. Estrogen doesn't just taper off gradually like a good girl. She can take us on an erratic, wild ride, so it can be frustrating to deal with a normal cycle sometimes and then wonder what's going on on Day 35 when your period is a no-show. You might go for a couple of months without a period, then start menstruating and feeling like you're back on track again, only to get another period on Day 12. What's up with that?

In addition to having the option to align with the moon cycle in between your menstrual cycles, this can also be a time when you call upon your mastery of energies, rhythms, and cycles. Find solace in circadian rhythms, doing what you can to settle yourself in for a good night's sleep each night. Experiment with portals—create your own time tunnels to work on special projects, or to take time to rest. Try a new-moon ritual each month to check in with your desires. Eat with the seasons. Take ultradian rhythm breaks throughout the day. There are always energy cycles and rhythms that you can leverage to support yourself. During perimenopause you get to practice energy-alignment flexibility. Do what works for you in each moment. If estrogen can make up her own rules, so can you!

Q: Can I manifest a particular person?

Rather than focusing on one particular person, whether it's a romantic partner, a new friend, or even a boss, it's best to shift your focus from that one individual to the *qualities* you truly want in a person. It can be tempting to fixate on one person, but remember that everyone has their own free will, and their path might not align with yours. Got a crush on a hottie? Try making a Love List of the traits you'd love a person to have, like kindness, honesty, ambition, or creativity. When you focus on these qualities, you're opening yourself up to the possibility of attracting the right people, whether they're already in your life or someone new. When you avoid fixating on a particular person, the Universe can bring the right connections your way and you will be more likely to recognize them. Manifesting around the qualities you desire creates space for something even better than you might have imagined. By trusting the process, honoring free will, and keeping your intentions open, you allow room for the right people to show up when the time is right.

Q: How do I know whether to take action or let go?

A large part of this journey is about developing your intuition. We've been so accustomed to operating in our masculine (logical) energy for so long that we can feel lost when we need to make an intuitive decision—we may inquire of others as to what they would do, or ask others to just decide for us. I invite you to take a moment of stillness, take a deep breath, and tune in to your inner knowing. Play out the scenario visualizing both options. Which felt better?

To explore further, consider which phase you're currently in. How would it feel to align with the predominant energy of that phase? If you're in Attune, you could go inward for answers; if in Awaken, you could take action if it feels right; if in Thrive, you could act with boldness and confidence; and if in Surrender, you could let go.

Ultimately, you will have to deal with the consequences of your decision, so choose the path that feels more aligned with how you wish to manage your energy. Consider whether taking action aligns with your long-term goals and values, or if letting go will create space for something better to come into your life. Find a balance between listening to your intuition and being mindful of the outcomes you truly desire.

Q: Why wasn't I taught about cycles earlier?

Friend, I hear you! Although it's frustrating to have discovered the empowerment that comes with aligning with natural energy cycles at the time in my life when I am flirting with perimenopause, instead of reflecting on all those lost years of "going it alone," I am forever grateful that I experimented with cycles and was guided to share this knowledge. Yes, it's something we should have been taught in school, and yes, it's something that every woman deserves to know. The fact is that we are all hurtling through space and time on a giant rock and subject to the energies, magnetic fields, and planetary rhythms all around us at every moment. Women have a vastly different hormonal rhythm than men, yet there is a gender bias in medical research that feeds us health guidance from a "mini man's" perspective. A wave of change is coming, and we are on the brink of it, but it can be challenging in the meantime to try to fit ourselves into a structure of living that doesn't align with a woman's natural way of being. It's okay to feel disturbed by this. Allow it to be fuel for the changes *you* will make in your own life. Feel into the gratitude over having discovered the magic of cycles when you did.

It's never too late to align with the moon cycle; she is always there for us. When we begin aligning with natural cycles, there's no stopping us. You can make up for that feeling of lost ground by getting started *now* and manifesting your dreams—whether it's marriage in your 40s, a 30-pound weight loss, healing from illness, living closer to the beach, building more wealth, acquiring certifications in a field that you love, creating your dream business, writing a book, or buying your dream car—all of which I have been able to manifest through my alignment with natural cycles in co-creation with the Universe in less than five years, even in the midst of a pandemic.

When it comes to the benefits of aligning with the moon cycle or the menstrual cycle, you can ask yourself in what ways you could pass this legacy on to others. Maybe by sharing the magic of cycles with a friend, sister, daughter, or niece? Learning to align with natural cycles is a gift of empowerment.

Congratulations, beautiful soul, for having the courage and faith to try a new approach to attract your dreams into reality. I wish you well on your journey and know that you have a unique light to shine in this world. You are well on your way to cycle mastery and becoming a co-creator with the Universe. I can't wait to see what *you* manifest! #CycleMagic

Love & Magic,
Elle

RESOURCES

Cycle Magic Tools

- Access your Heart and Soul Desires guided meditation audio download at CycleMagic.com/meditation.

- Visit CycleHabits.com/tracker to download your blank Cycle Habits Tracker sheet. Print the sheet, making as many copies as you like, or use the Cycle Habits Tracker digitally by opening the file after you downloaded it with a PDF annotation app such as Goodnotes or Canva on your tablet, phone, or computer.

- Become a Cycle Magic member and access monthly group coaching with Elle Serafina, topical master classes, a hormone health hub, Moonology forecasts, over 100 cycle-aligned recipes from The Cycle Diet collection, and more. Visit CycleMagic.com to join this community of like-minded women.

Cycle Apps and Trackers

- Clue app for menstrual cycle tracking: www.helloclue.com

- iPhone Health app Cycle Tracking function

- My Moon Phase lunar calendar app: www.jrustonapps.com/apps/my-moon-phase
- Natural Cycles menstrual cycle tracking: www.naturalcycles.com
- Oura Ring device and app: www.ouraring.com
- Rivolu desktop moon calendar: www.rivolu.com

Health and Wellness

- American College of Lifestyle Medicine: www.lifestylemedicine.org
- Blue Zones longevity: www.bluezones.com
- Equinox gym: www.equinox.com
- Goop clean beauty: www.goop.com
- Harvard Medical School Executive Education: https://learn.hms.harvard.edu/about/program-categories/executive-education
- HeartMath heart-brain coherence tools: www.heartmath.com
- HigherDOSE wellness products: www.higherdose.com
- Institute for Integrative Nutrition: www.integrativenutrition.com
- Kora Organics skin care: www.koraorganics.com
- Living Libations essential oils and beauty: www.livinglibations.com
- Medical Medium books and recipes: www.medicalmedium.com

- Melissa Wood Health: www.melissawoodhealth.com
- Pilates by Bryony: www.pilatesbybryony.com
- Pvolve workouts: www.pvolve.com
- Sakara meal delivery: www.sakara.com
- Therabody wellness technology: www.therabody.com
- Vimergy supplements: www.vimergy.com

Spirituality and Mindfulness
Books, courses, events, podcasts and more.
- Astrology Zone: www.astrologyzone.com
- Deepak Chopra www.deepakchopra.com
- Hay House: www.hayhouse.com
- Human Design: www.myhumandesign.com
- Insight Timer: www.insighttimer.com
- Kabbalah Centre: www.kabbalah.com
- Moonology: www.yasminboland.com

REFERENCES

Introduction

1. Marèn Hoogland and Annemie Ploeger, "Two Different Mismatches: Integrating the Developmental and the Evolutionary-Mismatch Hypothesis," *Perspectives on Psychological Science* 17, no. 6 (November 2022), https://pmc.ncbi.nlm.nih.gov/articles/PMC9634284.
2. Dan Witters, "U.S. Depression Rates Reach New Highs," Gallup, May 17, 2023, https://news.gallup.com/poll/505745/depression-rates-reach-new-highs.aspx.
3. Christine Kuehner, "Why Is Depression More Common Among Women Than Among Men?" *Lancet Psychiatry* 4, no. 2 (February 2017): 146–158, https://pubmed.ncbi.nlm.nih.gov/27856392. Anxiety and Depression Association of America, "Anxiety Disorders—Facts and Statistics," n.d., https://adaa.org/understanding-anxiety/facts-statistics.
4. "The Effects of Stress on Your Body," WebMD, February 29, 2024, https://www.webmd.com/balance/stress-management/effects-of-stress-on-your-body.

Chapter 1

1. Ruheea Taskin Ruhee and Katsuhiko Suzuki, "The Integrative Role of Sulforaphane in Preventing Inflammation, Oxidative Stress and Fatigue: A Review of a Potential Protective Phytochemical," *Antioxidants* (Basel) 9, no. 6 (June 13, 2020): 521, https://pmc.ncbi.nlm.nih.gov/articles/PMC7346151.
2. 1. P. B. Lissaman and C. A. Shollenberger, "Formation Flight of Birds," *Science* 168, no. 3934 (May 22, 1970): 1003–1005, https://pubmed.ncbi.nlm.nih.gov/5441020.

Chapter 2

1. Mihaly Csikszentmihalyi, "Preface," *Flow: The Psychology of Optimal Experience* (New York: Harper & Row, 1990), https://www.researchgate.net/publication/224927532_Flow_The_Psychology_of_Optimal_Experience.

2. David J. Handelsman, Angelica L. Hirschberg, and Stephane Bermon, "Circulating Testosterone as the Hormonal Basis of Sex Differences in Athletic Performance," *Endocrine Reviews* 39, no. 5 (July 13, 2018): 803–829, https://pmc.ncbi.nlm.nih.gov/articles/PMC6391653.

Chapter 4

1. "The Energetic Heart Is Unfolding," HeartMath Institute, July 22, 2010, https://www.heartmath.org/articles-of-the-heart/science-of-the-heart/the-energetic-heart-is-unfolding.

2. Clara Moskowitz, "Fact or Fiction? Energy Can Neither Be Created nor Destroyed," *Scientific American*, August 5, 2014, https://www.scientificamerican.com/article/energy-can-neither-be-created-nor-destroyed.

3. "Neuroplasticity 101," BrainFutures, accessed December 30, 2024, https://www.brainfutures.org/neuroplasticity-101.

4. Regina Pally, "The Predicting Brain: Unconscious Repetition, Conscious Reflection and Therapeutic Change," *The International Journal of Psycho-Analysis* 88, Part 4 (August 2007): 861–881, https://pubmed.ncbi.nlm.nih.gov/17681897.

5. "EEG Definitions," NeuroHealth, accessed December 30, 2024, https://nhahealth.com/brainwaves-the-language.

6. Gaétan Chevalier, et al., "Earthing: Health Implications of Reconnecting the Human Body to the Earth's Surface Electrons," *Journal of Environmental and Public Health* (January 12, 2012): 291541, https://pmc.ncbi.nlm.nih.gov/articles/PMC3265077.

7. "Microbiome," *Nature Reviews Microbiology*, https://www.nature.com/collections/stkpgwjvvk.

Chapter 5

1. Jeevan Kumar Gullari, "The Impact of Moon Phases on Earth, Plants, and Humans: A Comprehensive Study from Project Alpha" SSRN (January 09, 2025) https://papers.ssrn.com/sol3/papers.cfm?abstract_id=5090101.

2. Lea Merone, et al., "Sex Inequalities in Medical Research: A Systematic Scoping Review of the Literature," *Women's Health Reports* (New Rochelle, NY) 31, no. 3 (January 31, 2022): 49–59, https://pmc.ncbi.nlm.nih.gov/articles/PMC8812498.

3. S. K. Gupta, E. A. Lindemulder, and G. Sathyan, "Modeling of Circadian Testosterone in Healthy Men and Hypogonadal Men," *Journal of Clinical Pharmacology* 40, no. 7 (July 2000): 731–738, https://pubmed.ncbi.nlm.nih.gov/10883414.

4. Helen E. Scharfman and Neil J. MacLusky, "Estrogen–Growth Factor Interactions and Their Contributions to Neurological Disorders," *Headache* 48, Supplement 2 (July 2008): S77–S89, https://pmc.ncbi.nlm.nih.gov/articles/PMC2729400.

5. Wu Jeong Hwang, et al., "The Role of Estrogen Receptors and Their Signaling Across Psychiatric Disorders," *International Journal of Molecular Sciences* 22, no. 1 (December 31, 2020): 373, https://pmc.ncbi.nlm.nih.gov/articles/PMC7794990.

6. Rui Du, Ting Liang, and Guofang Lu, "Modulation of Empathic Abilities by the Interplay Between Estrogen Receptors and Arginine Vasopressin," *Neuroscience Research* 210 (January 2025): 11–18, https://www.sciencedirect.com/science/article/pii/S016801022400110X.

7. Marcus E. Raichle and Debra A. Gusnard, "Appraising the Brain's Energy Budget," *Proceedings of the National Academy of Sciences of the United States of America* 99, no. 16 (July 29, 2002): 10237–10239, https://pmc.ncbi.nlm.nih.gov/articles/PMC124895.

8. Nicole P. Bowles, et al., "The Circadian System Modulates the Cortisol Awakening Response in Humans," *Frontiers in Neuroscience* 16 (November 3, 2022): 995452, https://pmc.ncbi.nlm.nih.gov/articles/PMC9669756.

9. Lucy Brian, "Alcohol and Sleep," Sleep Foundation, updated July 16, 2025, https://www.sleepfoundation.org/nutrition/alcohol-and-sleep.

10. "The Health Benefits of Strong Relationships," Harvard Health Publishing, December 1, 2010, https://www.health.harvard.edu/staying-healthy/the-health-benefits-of-strong-relationships.
11. Manoj K. Bhasin, et al., "Specific Transcriptome Changes Associated with Blood Pressure Reduction in Hypertensive Patients After Relaxation Response Training," *Journal of Alternative and Complementary Medicine* 24, no. 5 (May 2018): 486–504, https://pubmed.ncbi.nlm.nih.gov/29616846.
12. Eric S. Kim, et al., "Association Between Purpose in Life and Objective Measures of Physical Function in Older Adults," *JAMA Psychiatry* 74, no. 10 (2017): 1039–1045, https://jamanetwork.com/journals/jamapsychiatry/fullarticle/2648692.
13. "Back to School: Learning a New Skill Can Slow Cognitive Aging," Harvard Health Publishing, April 27, 2016, https://www.health.harvard.edu/blog/learning-new-skill-can-slow-cognitive-aging-201604279502.
14. William R. Marchand, "Neural Mechanisms of Mindfulness and Meditation: Evidence from Neuroimaging Studies," *World Journal of Radiology* 6, no. 7 (July 28, 2014): 471–479, https://pmc.ncbi.nlm.nih.gov/articles/PMC4109098.
15. Ghalia M. Attia, Ohood A. Alharbi, and Reema M. Aljohani, "The Impact of Irregular Menstruation on Health: A Review of the Literature," *Cureus* 15, no. 11 (November 20, 2023): e49146, https://pmc.ncbi.nlm.nih.gov/articles/PMC10733621.
16. "Understanding Thyroid Problems & Disease," Weill Cornell Medicine, January 25, 2022, https://weillcornell.org/news/understanding-thyroid-problems-disease#.

Chapter 6

1. C. Helfrich-Förster, et al., "Women Temporarily Synchronize Their Menstrual Cycles with the Luminance and Gravimetric Cycles of the Moon," *Science Advances* 7, no. 5 (January 27, 2021), https://www.science.org/doi/10.1126/sciadv.abe1358.
2. Christian Cajochen, et al., "Evidence That the Lunar Cycle Influences Human Sleep," *Current Biology* 23, no. 15 (August 5, 2013): 1485–1488, https://pubmed.ncbi.nlm.nih.gov/23891110.

3. Weizmann Institute of Science, "Quantum Theory Demonstrated: Observation Affects Reality," February 27, 1998, *Science Daily*, https://www.sciencedaily.com/releases/1998/02/980227055013.htm.

4. "Science of the Heart: Exploring the Role of the Heart in Human Performance," HeartMath Institute, accessed December 30, 2024, https://www.heartmath.org/research/science-of-the-heart/energetic-communication.

Chapter 7

1. Celine Bencker, et al., "Progestagens and Progesterone Receptor Modulation: Effects on the Brain, Mood, Stress, and Cognition in Females," *Frontiers in Neuroendocrinology* 76 (January 2025): 101160, https://www.sciencedirect.com/science/article/pii/S0091302224000402.

2. Sabrina K. Syan, et al., "Influence of Endogenous Estradiol, Progesterone, Allopregnanolone, and Dehydroepiandrosterone Sulfate on Brain Resting State Functional Connectivity Across the Menstrual Cycle," *Fertility and Sterility* 107, no. 5 (May 2017): 1246–1255, https://pubmed.ncbi.nlm.nih.gov/28476183.

3. Malgorzata Stefaniak, et al., "Progesterone and Its Metabolites Play a Beneficial Role in Affect Regulation in the Female Brain," *Pharmaceuticals* (Basel) 16, no. 4 (March 31, 2023): 520, https://pmc.ncbi.nlm.nih.gov/articles/PMC10143192.

4. Leszek A. Rybaczyk, et al., "An Overlooked Connection: Serotonergic Mediation of Estrogen-Related Physiology and Pathology," *BMC Women's Health* 5 (December 20, 2005): 12, https://pmc.ncbi.nlm.nih.gov/articles/PMC1327664.

5. Jonathan Shaw, "Born to Rest," *Harvard Magazine*, September–October 2016, https://www.harvardmagazine.com/2016/08/born-to-rest; Benjamin C. Trumble, et al., "Energetic Costs of Testosterone in Two Subsistence Populations," *American Journal of Human Biology* 35, no. 11 (November 2023): e23949, https://pubmed.ncbi.nlm.nih.gov/37365845.

6. Georges Copinschi, Fred W. Turek, and Eve Van Cauter, "Chapter 11: Endocrine Rhythms, the Sleep-Wake Cycle, and Biological Clocks," in *Endocrinology: Adult and Pediatric*, ed. J. Larry Jameson

and Leslie J. De Groot, vol. 1 (Philadelphia: Saunders, 2010), pp. 199–229, https://www.sciencedirect.com/science/article/abs/pii/B9781416055839000113?via=ihub.

7. Janine Thome, et al., "Back to the Basics: Resting State Functional Connectivity of the Reticular Activation System in PTSD and Its Dissociative Subtype," *Chronic Stress* (Thousand Oaks) 3 (September 27, 2019): 2470547019873663, https://pmc.ncbi.nlm.nih.gov/articles/PMC7219926.

ABOUT THE AUTHOR

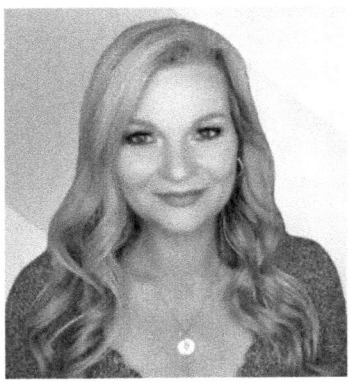

Intuitive Wellness Coach **Elle Serafina** supports women to manifest more ease and flow in their lives by tapping in to their innate energies and natural cycles. As a certified Integrative Nutrition Health Coach specializing in hormone health, Elle studied holistic lifestyle medicine approaches at Harvard Medical School and the Institute for Integrative Nutrition. Through more than two decades of spiritual study and practice, Elle has honed her empathic and intuitive gifts by becoming a certified Moonologer and Law of Attraction practitioner. Drawing upon her passions for spirituality and feminine energy, she created the Cycle Magic® system for women to manifest their heart and soul desires, the Cycle Habits® Tracker for goal achievement, and The Cycle Diet® recipe collection, helping women balance their hormones naturally. Elle lives with her husband and two kitties in Orange County, California. Find Elle online at **ElleSerafina.com** or **CycleMagic.com** and her social media channels.

CONNECT WITH ELLE

- Facebook @page.ElleSerafina
- Instagram @Elle.Serafina
- LinkedIn @Elle-Serafina
- Pinterest @ElleSerafina
- TikTok @Elle_Serafina
- X @Elle_Serafina
- YouTube @ElleSerafina

#CycleMagic #CycleHabits #TheCycleDiet #Misaligned #MeantForMore

ACKNOWLEDGMENTS

Beloved reader, crafting this book has brought me so much joy because I've had YOU in mind throughout the entire process. I've conversed with the Creator each day over the past two years while weaving this content together, with the intention that these words uplift you to feel empowered to live a life you love and radiate your unique light in the world. Thank you for allowing me the opportunity to walk alongside you on this journey and share my discoveries with you. May your heart and soul desires unfold with ease.

I've always sensed a structure within the unseen forces of this world, though I didn't truly understand it until I discovered the spiritual wisdom of Kabbalah 20 years ago, and I've been a student ever since. To Michael and Monica Berg, thank you for instilling in me the belief that we all carry a spark of light inside us that holds a power far beyond what we can comprehend. Thank you for embodying what it means to lead with certainty, compassion, and authenticity. With deep love and gratitude to my Kabbalah Centre family.

Receiving a call from Reid Tracy welcoming me to the Hay House family remains one of the highlights of my life. I am truly humbled to be among such visionary authors, continuing the compassionate work of Louise Hay. Anthony William, thank you for your words of encouragement, you have touched my soul, and you are a healing force in my life. Heartfelt thanks to my editor, Sally Mason-Swaab, for your encouragement, patience, and wisdom, and for guiding me through this journey. Deep gratitude to the Hay House team, with a special shout-out to the Creative Team for bringing my cover design vision to life, and to Charlie Griffin for your generosity and expertise.

To Kelly Notaras and Jill Esplin of KN Literary Arts, thank you for sharing your knowledge, and connecting me with the perfect book proposal editor. Audra Figgins, I can't thank you enough for your insightful questions, prompts, and guidance. You helped me find clarity, and the confidence to know that I could do this!

Deep gratitude to Dr. Beth Frates, Harvard Medical School physician and pioneer in Lifestyle Medicine. You've taught me that wellness can be simple, and that we all have the tools to support our health through mindful lifestyle choices. May your message inspire millions around the world. I'm grateful to Joshua Rosenthal and the teachers at the Institute for Integrative Nutrition for trailblazing holistic health and empowering countless individuals to become catalysts for wellness. Your teachings have illuminated the path to balanced living and shaped my own approach to natural health and hormone harmony.

Appreciation to Yasmin Boland for your Moonology teachings, which have deepened my connection to the cycles of the moon and feminine energy. To Dr. Joe Vitale, thank you for your guidance on the principles of the Law of Attraction, which have inspired and influenced how I approach conscious creation and manifestation.

Heartfelt gratitude to my coaching clients and Cycle Magic members whose dedication to living a life of wellness continually inspires me. Thank you to Mary Shaughnessy for your financial expertise, and to Karima Gulick and team for your legal guidance. Appreciation to Susie Moore and team for publicity and media support.

To my wonderful friends, I am so grateful for your patience and love as I worked on this special project behind the scenes. Linda, Sandra, Leah, thank you for believing in me. Thank you to my soul sister, Georgia Papadimitri, for your unwavering love and support.

To my family, my biggest supporters, thank you for your patience and well wishes throughout this process. Sherry, Dennis, Shila, Arman, Christina and Afshar—words can't express how much you've brightened my life. It's an honor to call you family. Thank you for bearing with me as I skipped Thanksgiving to journey through a writing portal, and for cheering me on over FaceTime and in real life. To my husband, Andre, as half the letters on my keyboard slowly faded away you've been the steady force in my life, always encouraging me. Thank you for holding the belief that I can do anything. To my darling kitties, Arabella Bijou and Leonardo Buxley, your presence fills our home with joy every day. Thank you for being my faithful writing buddies. Dad, I know you would feel so proud that I wrote a book. Thank you for always caring about my well-being and for being a catalyst for change in my life. To my nan, Olive May, thank you for your unconditional love, kindness, and constant companionship. You helped shape me into who I am today.

Disclaimer: This book provides general information and discussion about wellness, health and related subjects. It is not intended and should not be construed as medical advice. If the reader or any other person has a medical concern, they should consult with an appropriately licensed physician or other health care worker. Elle Serafina is not a licensed medical doctor or other formally licensed health care professional, and does not render medical, psychological, or other professional advice or treatment, nor provide or prescribe any medical diagnosis, treatment, medication, or remedy. The information provided is for informational purposes only and should not be considered to be health care advice or medical diagnosis, treatment or prescribing. None of this information should be considered a promise of benefits, a claim of cures, a legal warranty or a guarantee of results to be achieved. This information is not intended as a substitute for advice from your physician or other health care professionals. You should consult with a health care professional before starting any diet, exercise, or supplementation program, or if you have or suspect you might have a health problem. The United States Food and Drug Administration has not evaluated any statement, claim, or representation made in this publication, or evaluated any food, product, or service mentioned. No food, product, or service mentioned is intended to diagnose, treat, cure, or prevent disease.

Hay House Titles of Related Interest

YOU CAN HEAL YOUR LIFE, the movie,
starring Louise Hay & Friends
(available as an online streaming video)
www.hayhouse.co.uk/louise-movie

THE SHIFT, the movie,
starring Dr Wayne W. Dyer
(available as an online streaming video)
www.hayhouse.co.uk/the-shift-movie

***

ACTIVATE YOUR FUTURE SELF: The Secret to Effortlessly Becoming the Happiest, Healthiest and Wealthiest You, by Mimi Bouchard

DO LESS: A Revolutionary Approach to Time and Energy Management for Ambitious Women, by Kate Northrup

THE LET THEM THEORY: A Life-Changing Tool That Millions of People Can't Stop Talking About, by Mel Robbins

SELF HELP: This Is Your Chance to Change Your Life, by Gabrielle Bernstein

All of the above are available at your local bookstore, or may be ordered by visiting:

Hay House UK: www.hayhouse.co.uk
Hay House USA: www.hayhouse.com®
Hay House Australia: www.hayhouse.com.au
Hay House India: www.hayhouse.co.in

We hope you enjoyed this Hay House book. If you'd like to receive our online catalogue featuring additional information on Hay House books and products, please contact:

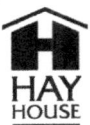

Hay House UK Ltd
1st Floor, Crawford Corner,
91–93 Baker Street, London W1U 6QQ
Tel: +44 (0)20 3927 7290; www.hayhouse.co.uk

Published in the United States of America by:
Hay House LLC
PO Box 5100, Carlsbad, CA 92018-5100
Tel: (760) 431-7695 or (800) 654-5126
www.hayhouse.com

Published in Australia by:
Hay House Australia Publishing Pty Ltd
18/36 Ralph St., Alexandria NSW 2015
Tel: +61 (02) 9669 4299
www.hayhouse.com.au

Published in India by:
Hay House Publishers (India) Pvt Ltd
Muskaan Complex, Plot No. 3,
B-2, Vasant Kunj, New Delhi 110 070
Tel: +91 11 41761620
www.hayhouse.co.in

Let Your Soul Grow

Experience life-changing transformation – one video at a time – with guidance from the world's leading experts.

www.healyourlifeplus.com

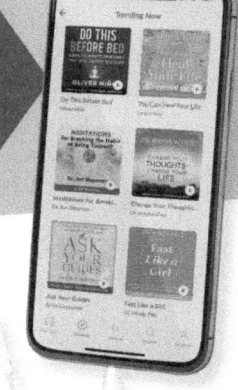

HAY HOUSE
Online Video Courses

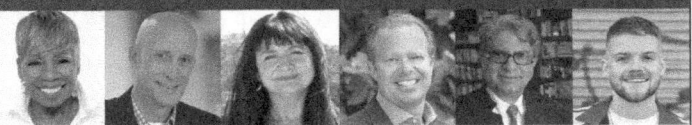

Your journey to a better life starts with figuring out which path is best for you. Hay House Online Courses provide guidance in mental and physical health, personal finance, telling your unique story, and so much more!

LEARN HOW TO:

- choose your words and actions wisely so you can tap into life's magic
- clear the energy in yourself and your environments for improved clarity, peace, and joy
- forgive, visualize, and trust in order to create a life of authenticity and abundance
- manifest lifelong health by improving nutrition, reducing stress, improving sleep, and more
- create your own unique angelic communication toolkit to help you to receive clear messages for yourself and others
- use the creative power of the quantum realm to create health and well-being

To find the guide for your journey, visit www.HayHouseU.com.

HAY HOUSE
online learning

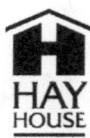

CONNECT WITH
HAY HOUSE
ONLINE

🌐 hayhouse.co.uk   **f** @hayhouse

📷 @hayhouseuk   🦋 @hayhouseuk.bsky.social

♪ @hayhouseuk   ▶ @HayHousePresents

Find out all about our latest books & card decks • Be the first to know about exclusive discounts • Interact with our authors in live broadcasts • Celebrate the cycle of the seasons with us • Watch free videos from your favourite authors • Connect with like-minded souls

'The gateways to wisdom and knowledge are always open.'

Louise Hay